Michel Montignac

Eat Yourself SLIM

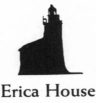

Erica House

BALTIMORE   AMSTERDAM   SALAMANCA

First printing

Translated from French by Erin Goodwillie.

ISBN: 1-893162-05-2
Library of Congress Catalog Card Number: 99-61527

PUBLISHED BY ERICA HOUSE BOOK PUBLISHERS
www.ericahouse.com

Baltimore   Amsterdam   Salamanca

Printed in the United States of America

TABLE OF CONTENTS

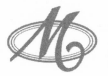

TABLE OF CONTENTS

PREAMBLE

All epidemological studies show that obesity is constantly rising in industrialized countries, despite a paradoxical decrease in caloric intake based on the recommended daily allowance.

For years, scientists had noted that in all forms of obesity, the same anomolies appeared in the secretion of a hormone, insulin, which was also implicated in diabetes, arterial hypertension and heart disease. But this hyperinsulinism (as well as insulinoresistance, which is the resulting complication) were instead considered a consequence of obesity.

Michel Montignac has always had the opposite hypothesis. Since his first books, he has expressed the idea that hyperinsulinism was, in fact, the cause of obesity and that its debilitating effects could result in well-known cardio-vascular complications.

Tracing the torrent of casualties, Michel Montignac stressed that this hyperinsulinism was the consequence of a more and more hyperglycemic modern diet, meaning principally composed of high-glycemic index carbohydrates (refined grains, potatoes, sugar...).

By advising the eating of low-glycemic index carbohydrates to the overweight, he obtained, with the decrease in the insulin response, a loss of weight as well as a reduction of risk factors (glycemia, triglycerides, cholesterol...).

For years, faced with Montignac's success, his critics enjoyed saying of his Method that it had never been scientifically proven.

Thus, the Canadian study conducted by Professor Dumesnil made public at the Congrès International de Paris in 1998 showed that the Montignac Method was more effective for weight loss than traditional diets and that it could prevent the factors of cardio-vascular risk.

The hypotheses that have been raised and defended for more than ten years by Michel Montignac have also been confirmed today by world-renowned scientific research like that of Professor Willet from the United States (*Science et Avenir*, February 1999).

Michel Montignac, long mocked and denigrated, is now seeing his theories affirmed by unquestionable scientific studies.

I am obviously thrilled to see the ideas which I have personally always believed triumph. But let us hope that in the mediatic storm surrounding this challenge to classic dietetics, it will not be forgotten that Michel Montignac was one of the pioneers of this great nutritional transformation of the third millenium.

Dr. Hervé Robert
Nutritional Doctor
Professor at the Faculté de Paris

PREFACE

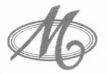

It is through personal experience that I first became acquainted with the Montignac Method. I was 52 years old and overweight (5ft. 7 in., 195 lb.). A friend and colleague of mine had been suggesting to me for some time that I buy this book (the French version of *Eat Yourself Slim*) by someone named Michel Montignac. He said he had discovered this new Method, which was different from traditional diets in that it did not advocate any restriction in quantity but was mainly based on a different selection of nutrients. He was very enthusiastic because he had lost a lot of weight, definitely felt better, and had been maintaining his ideal weight for quite some time without any difficulty.

I must confess that I was skeptical at first. I had followed other diets in the past. As is the case with many people, I had initially lost weight but had later regained more than I had lost. The main reason for these failures was a profound sense of deprivation arising from the continued necessity to restrict food intake in order to maintain weight loss. In none of these attempts had I lost more than 20 pounds, let alone attained my ideal weight.

The true revelation came when my wife and I went to a reception with my friend and saw what they were eating. My wife bought the book the next day, and the rest, as they say, is history. I immediately started losing weight to the tune of three to five pounds a week in the beginning and then more slowly. At the end of six months, I had lost 45 pounds without much difficulty, and I was feeling great.

Being a cardiologist and researcher, I was also very curious as to why the Method worked so well and wondered if it could not be applied with success on a more widespread basis. Obesity is reaching near endemic proportions in North America (based on World Health Organization definitions, close to 50% of the population is either obese or overweight). The consequences are potentially devastating from the standpoint of diseases such as diabetes and cardiovascular disorders. Yet the treatment of obesity has been very discouraging, if not completely unsuccessful. Drugs such as fen-phen have been used with some success but had to be withdrawn because of unacceptable side effects. Considering the high prevalence of obesity and its progression, the administration of drugs to such a wide segment of the population also appears somewhat unnatural (taking drugs in order to be able to eat) as well as prohibitive from an economic standpoint. As for traditional diets, their success rate for long-term maintenance of weight loss is very low (less than 5% compared to 15-20% for programs designed to stop smoking or drinking alcohol). Then, here was this new Method with which it was relatively easy to lose weight in significant and unprecedented proportions without really being hungry or feeling deprived.

It is in this context that colleagues of mine, two of whom had successfully followed the Method, and myself contacted colleagues of ours at Laval University who are renowned experts in nutrition and the epidemiology of lipid disorders. They were surprised by our queries, but given our enthusiasm and willingness to advance funding, they agreed that it might be worthwhile to do a pilot study, and a protocol was drafted.

The study thus included twelve overweight men who were submitted to three six-day regimens during which all meals were taken in the hospital. Food intake was measured meticulously in terms of calories and macro-nutrients (carbohydrates, lipids and proteins), and blood samples were taken before and after each regimen to measure parameters such as blood sugar, insulin, cholesterol and other lipid fractions.

The first week consisted of a low fat diet based on the recommendations of the American Heart Association with no restriction on the quantity of food to be consumed. The second week, they followed the Montignac Method, also with no restriction on the quantity of food to be consumed. In the third week, they were given the same number of calories they had taken in during the second week, but with the same macro-nutrient composition as in the first week. Also, the subjects were administered standardized questionnaires asking them to rate their hunger and degree of satiety before and after each meal.

At the end of the study, we were amazed at the results. During the Montignac week, the subjects had spontaneously eaten less than during the first week, but without being hungrier or feeling deprived. In contrast, during the third week, where they had eaten the same number of calories as during the Montignac week they felt much more hungry and deprived, to the extent that some of them even wanted to leave the study. Moreover, they lost slightly more weight during the Montignac week than during the third week, and beneficial effects on their blood lipids and fasting insulin levels were observed only during the Montignac week.

The Method proposed by Monsieur Montignac, based on choosing carbohydrates exclusively from among foods with a low glycemic index is therefore very interesting from many standpoints. First, there is no doubt that it works very well for losing weight. Second, because it is relatively easy to follow and has neutral effects on hunger and satiety, it offers more hope than conventional low calorie diets for the long-term maintenance of weight loss. One must remember that most diets fail in the long term because of a continued sensation of deprivation and hunger.

Finally, our results also suggest that the Montignac Method has unique beneficial effects on blood lipids and fasting insulin levels, and in the new edition, further attention is given to the prevention of hypercholesterolemia and cardiovascular disorders (Chapter 8). For these reasons, we think the Montignac Method is full of promise, and we intend to continue to investigate the mechanisms underlying its efficacy as well as its potential long-term beneficial effects on disorders such as diabetes and cardiovascular diseases.

As far as I am personally concerned, I have now been following the Method for two years, I am still feeling great, and I am maintaining the same weight without any difficulty.

Jean G. Dumesnil, MD, FRCP, FACC,
Cardiologist, Quebec Heart Institute, Laval Hospital,
Professor of Medicine and Director, Cardiology Training Program

FOREWORD

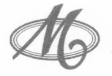

Excessive weight and, *a fortiori*, obesity are social phenomena. In a way, they are by-products of civilization. Primitive societies generally do not have a problem with obesity. Similarly, obesity is non-existent in the animal kingdom for species living in their natural environments. Only animals domesticated by humans show the symptoms of it.

Paradoxically, excessive weight problems are worst in the most evolved societies. In effect, it seems that obesity directly corresponds to people's standards of living. Moreover, we have been able to observe this phenomenon throughout the course of history. With few exceptions, the most overweight individuals have been associated with the wealthiest social categories. Being overweight was usually considered a virtue. It was not only a symbol of social success, but also of good health. Have we not referred to overweight people as "robust"?

Today's mentalities have evolved because, aside from the fact that the canons of beauty have changed, we have progressively become aware of the ravages of excess weight. Obesity is now considered a danger because we know that it is an important risk factor when it comes to health. If we were to examine the state of obesity around the world, we would find it most catastrophic in the United States, although it is reaching comparable levels in a number of other countries, notably Russia. Considering the American diet, it is easy to see that poor eating habits are at the heart of obesity, which becomes worse every year. But obesity is also appearing at a frightening rate in all of the countries where American eating styles have been exported.

Contrary to what certain practitioners too-frequently suggest, obesity is not a result of fate. Its origins are quite often hereditary, but this does not lessen the fact that all obesity comes from poor eating habits. Discussing the topic without recognizing this important point would be concentrating on the effect (the weight) while neglecting the cause. This reductionist approach is the downfall of traditional dietetics. Instead of looking to fad diets to lose pounds, we would do better to intelligently analyze why we gain weight. Instead of blindly following lists of ready-made menus, counting calories or measuring food, we would do better to try to understand how our body functions and in what ways it assimilates different types of food.

The process of losing weight and keeping it off begins with an obligatory educative phase. Before beginning to put the principles described in this book into action, I invite you to go over three steps that will help you to become knowledgeable about the topic. Knowledgeable, first of all, about the deplorable eating habits we have acquired over several decades, which can be associated with the consumption of refined food, and whose consequence is the progressive destabilization of our metabolism. This is what causes obesity and poor health. Knowledgeable, next, about the way our body functions. In effect, we must learn how metabolism and the digestive system operate. Knowledgeable, finally, about the nature of food, its properties and the families to which it belongs.

With this knowledge, you will be able to concretely construct an intelligent nutritional program that will give you the means to take charge of yourself and learn not only to manage your diet, but also to manage your weight for good. I invite you to discover all of this in the following chapters.

INTRODUCTION

Over the last few years, every time I was asked how I have stayed thin, I answered, "by eating in restaurants and by going to business dinners." It made people smile, but didn't really convince them. Undoubtedly it seems paradoxical, especially if you attribute your own heaviness to family, social, and perhaps professional obligations that lead you to honor - a little too often - the gastronomy of your country.

Most likely, you have already tried an infinite number of the popular diets that have been considered commonplace for a long time. Nevertheless, you may have noticed that the methods often contradict each other and produce temporary, if any, results. Moreover, you may have found it practically impossible to fit these diets into the framework of your normal lifestyle. Even at home they present so many constraints that they are quickly discouraging. Thus you are just as concerned today as you were a few years ago by what we will modestly call your excess weight.

For me, as for many of you, being overweight was a constant concern for many years. At eight years old, I was already much too fat. My father was obese and the men in my family weighed, for the most part, much over average. Thus, during my pre-adolescence I suffered a great deal from being fatter than my little friends. They did not hold back from making jokes about my pudginess, pouring out not-so-flattering qualifiers.

In the years that followed I was lucky enough to grow tall very quickly, which translated into a break in my weight-gain. But as soon as I turned 25, the extra pounds progressively reappeared, despite constant exercise and the restrictions I placed on myself at the time. Ten years later, on the eve of the 1980s, I was rather critically overweight - by twenty-five pounds. And then, from one day to the next, my professional situation evolved and I had to work in completely different conditions. I was given an international post at the heart of the general European division of a large American pharmaceutical company. From then on I traveled all the time, and my visits to the subsidiaries of which I was in charge were invariably inclined to have meetings centered on food.

Back in Paris I had to accompany visitors, for the most part foreigners, to the best French restaurants in the capital because of my duties with internal public relations. This was part of my professional obligation, and I must say it wasn't the most disagreeable part of my job. But three months after having taken on my new responsibilities, I had gained eleven pounds. I have to admit that during this period I had given a three-week course in England, which didn't help matters at all.

The alarm was sounding. My situation was becoming urgent.

Like everyone with weight problems, I tried applying the usual dietetic advice consisting of reducing energy supply (especially fats) and continuing to do physical exercise. The results were naturally most disappointing.

And then, on the occasion of a long trip to the United States and some good luck, I met some nutrition researchers who did not at all share the traditional dietetic point of view but did not propose other alternatives either. Amused by my desire (quasi-obsessive) to find a solution to my weight problem, they gave me access to a library full of hundreds of scientific studies conducted on the subject.

It was in exploring the diverse works published on diabetes that I discovered the path that would put me on the right track. The studies showed that 80% of diabetics were also obese. One could therefore imagine that the two pathologies had a common origin. Because the experiments had shown that by consuming exclusively carbohydrates with a weak glycemic potential, type II diabetics (non-insulin dependent) had substantially improved (even suppressed) their diabetes.

All I had to do, then, was try this nutritional approach to see if it could have a positive effect on weight loss. The result was spectacular. In very little time, I had lost a promising amount of weight. So I decided to delve more deeply into the matter, which was relatively easy for me to do since I worked in the field of science.

In a few months, I had lost a total of 35 pounds by eating normally, meaning without quantitative restriction but by, on the other hand, making particular choices among foods. In addition, frequently eating in restaurants made it even easier for me because as soon as you have a menu in front of you, you are inevitably in an ideal situation in terms of choice.

By reading this book, you will come to understand how I was thus able to permanently eliminate a very serious weight problem by my mere choice of food, without any restriction in terms of quantity and without obligation to do supplementary physical exercise.

After a few months, I compiled for my colleagues - and at their request - the essentials of the nutritional Method that I had developed and which took up three typed pages. They continually harassed me with questions. Everyone wanted to know how I was able to come up with this miracle - losing weight by eating. I tried, as much as possible, to spend one hour with each interested person to explain the basic principles of the Method. But that was not always sufficient. The foolish mistakes that were accidentally made too often compromised the results. In any case, the cultural power of generally accepted ideas, in total contradiction with my new nutritional principles, was too much and made the understanding of them ambiguous. The necessity to write a more complete document developed in my mind.

This book is a guide, and in writing it, I was seeking to leave you with the following objectives:

- to demystify generally accepted ideas by a sufficiently convincing argumentation so that they will be definitively abandoned,

- to provide fundamental scientific bases, indispensable to the comprehension of the metabolic phenomena that affect weight gain,

- to lay out simple rules and to provide the essentials of their technical and scientific validity,

- to reveal all the conditions of the Method's application in the tiniest detail, and

- to give, as much as possible, a veritable methodology - to make somewhat of a practical guide of this book.

For the past few years, with the advice of professionals, I have observed, researched, tested, and experimented. Today I feel confident that I have discovered and elaborated on an effective and easy method to put into practice.

You will learn in this book that we don't gain weight because we eat too much, but because we eat poorly. You will learn to manage your food intake just as one manages a budget. You will learn to balance your family, social, and professional obligations with your personal pleasure. Finally, you will learn to eat better without being unhappy.

But this book does not outline a "diet." It describes a new method of eating that consists of learning to maintain your ideal weight while continuing to profit from the pleasures of the table, whether you are at home, at a friend's home, or in a restaurant. You will be pleasantly surprised to learn that by adopting these new nutritional principles, you will find, as if by magic, a physical and intellectual vitality that you thought you had lost long ago. And I will tell you why.

You will learn that quite often certain nutritional habits are at the root of your lack of fitness and, consequentially, of athletic under-performance. You will understand that by adopting a few fundamental nutritional principles that are easy to put into practice, you will be able to end your midday slumps and discover optimal vitality. That is why, even in cases where you are barely or not at all overweight, learning and adopting the Method and its principles is still important for developing good diet management.

In any case, you will discover a new energy, the guarantee of better efficiency in all the tasks of your personal and professional life. You will also notice that the gastrointestinal problems you thought you were destined to live with will disappear completely because your digestive system will have been completely re-balanced.

Although I do praise good French cuisine in general, wine and chocolate in particular, in this book, it was definitely not my intention to plagiarize one of the excellent gastronomic guides that you are all familiar with. Just the same, I confess to sometimes having been tempted to do so because it has been difficult for me to dissociate nourishment from pleasure and simple cooking from gastronomical cuisine. For a few years I was lucky enough to frequent the best restaurants in the world, and the handshake of a great chef inspired in me respect and admiration.

Note:

The first version of this book came out in France in 1987. At that time, not a single editor would publish it. The fact that its author was unknown and that the book's contents totally challenged the theory of official dietetics did not reassure them.

Thus this book was first published "at the author's expense". Since it was not distributed in bookstores, it was only sold by correspondence. But since each book sold led to the sale of a dozen more, after four years by word of mouth a million copies had been sold. A little more than ten years later, more than five million copies had been sold in France and seven million worldwide. Today, this book has been published in 25 countries and translated into 18 languages.

Since the publication of this book, its nutritional message has been enriched and refined, not only from the testimonies of thousands of readers, but from the observations made by a great number of doctors who prescribe the Method. During all these years, I have personally dedicated most of my time and revenue to pursuing these research efforts so as to present an even clearer message. The systematic criticisms of opponents of all kinds have helped me a great deal in the sense that, despite the evidence of the efficacy of my Method, I have been forced to elaborate on its scientific bases. Not only can we refer to the observations of hundreds of researchers in their scientific publications (see bibliography) but also we can rely on specific studies on the Montignac Method whose positive results go beyond anything we had hoped for.

CHAPTER 1

Chapter 1

THE CALORIE MYTH

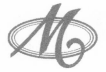

The idea of basing weight loss on a low-calorie diet is definitely the biggest scientific drivel of the twentieth century. It's a trap, a deception, a simplistic and dangerous "hypothesis," without real scientific foundation.   Yet it has governed our nutritional conduct for more than half a century.   Look around, and you'll notice that the more people are chubby, fat, or even obese, the more they relentlessly count the calories they take in. Except for a few rare exceptions, everything that we've called a "diet" since the beginning of the century has essentially been based on cutting calories.

Wrongly so! No serious long-term weight loss is possible using that method, not to mention the dangerous side effects that can occur. Never will we be able to denounce strongly enough this scandalous socio-cultural phenomenon that has developed around calories. To call it honest-to-goodness "collective conditioning" at this current stage is not an exaggeration.

ORIGIN OF THE CALORIE THEORY

In 1930, two American doctors from the University of Michigan published their idea that obesity was the result of a diet too "rich" in calories, more so than that of a metabolism deficiency. They directed a study on the balance of energy, which, in fact, was based on a very limited number of observations. But even more importantly, the time period over which it was conducted was much too brief to provide for a serious scientific foundation.

Despite this, the results were welcomed, as soon as they were published, as irrefutable, scientific truth, and they have since been considered a "gospel" of sorts. Yet some years later the two researchers, without a doubt troubled by the fuss made over their discovery, quietly showed some serious reservations about the conclusions that had made them so successful. But that went completely unseen. Their theory was already inscribed into the medical school curriculums of most western countries, and still today, it holds its own.

THE CALORIE THEORY: AN ILLUSION

A calorie is the amount of energy necessary to raise the temperature of one gram of water from 14 to 15 degrees Celsius. First of all, the human body needs energy to maintain a temperature of 98.6 degrees Fahrenheit; in some ways this is its primary need. But the moment the body becomes active, even if it is only to maintain an upright position, to move about, or to express sounds, a supplementary energy need is introduced. And then in order to eat, digest, and accomplish everyday movements, we again need more energy. But daily energy needs vary among individuals, ages and genders.

The calorie theory is the following:

If the energy needs of an individual are, for example, 2500 calories a day, and he or she only takes in 2000, a 500-calorie deficit will be created. In order to compensate this, the human body will take an amount of energy equal to the deficit from stored fats, which will consequently lead to weight loss. On the other hand, if an individual consumes 3500 calories daily, even though he or she only needs 2500, that person will create an excess of 1000 calories that will automatically be stored in the form of fat.

The theory, then, is derived from the postulate that states that, no matter what, energy can neither be created nor destroyed. It's mathematical. The formula comes from an equation that is directly inspired from Lavoisier's theory on thermodynamic laws.

At this point one might begin to ask how prisoners of concentration camps were able to survive for nearly five years with only 700 to 800 calories a day. If the calorie theory were true, the prisoners should have died after just a few months, having already used up their fatty and muscular masses.

In the same way, one could ask why some people who take in 4000 to 5000 calories a day don't weigh more (some always stay thin). If the calorie theory is true, these individuals should weigh 900 to 1000 pounds at the end just a few years.

How does one explain, on the other hand, that by eating less and, therefore, reducing the recommended number of consumed calories, certain people continue to gain weight? Millions of these individuals gain weight while, even though they are starving themselves.

THE CALORIC PARADOX

The first question is why, in reducing our calorie intake, can we not lose weight? In fact, weight loss does occur, but it is temporary. And this is, in reality, the reason for which the researchers from the University of Michigan were mistaken. Their observations were, in effect, based on an observation time that was much too brief.

The process goes like this:

Let's again assume that an individual's recommended needs are at 2500 calories and that, over an extended period of time, a supply of calories is designed according to those needs. If suddenly the ration of calories drops to 2000, the body will, as a result, use up a quantity of stored fats equal to the deficit, and we will be able to see weight loss.

On the other hand, if the subject then establishes his or her supply of calories at 2000 instead of the original 2500, the body, moved by its survival instinct, will very rapidly adjust its energy needs to the level of the supply. Now that it is only being provided with 2000 calories, it will only consume 2000. Weight loss, therefore, will be rapidly interrupted.

But the body's response won't stop there. Its survival instinct will push for greater caution, so much so that it will create reserves. If, from then on, it is provided with only 2000 calories, well then, it will again cut back its energy needs to, for example, 1700 and then store the 300-calorie difference as fat reserves.

Thus we get the inverse result of the one we were counting on because paradoxically, even though our subject is eating less, he or she is going to progressively gain the weight back. In fact, the human being, unfailingly moved by his or her survival instinct, behaves no differently than a dog that buries its bones even though it is starving. Ironically, it is as soon as the dog is fed on an irregular basis that it calls on its instincts and buries its food, building up reserves even though it's starving.

Furthermore, we must acknowledge that calculations of calories are always theoretical and even approximate for the following reasons:

- From one chart or table to the next, the calorie-count for a single food can vary substantially.
- The caloric content of some foods fluctuates based on whether the foods are eaten raw or cooked, with or without added fats.
- Fat content (which causes the caloric content to vary) can fluctuate a great deal, from one piece of meat to the other. The fluctuation is dependent upon the way the animal was raised as well as the method in which it was cooked.
- The calculation (theoretical) of calories never takes into consideration the rate of absorption of lipids and carbohydrates by the small intestine. This rate varies significantly based on the extent to which fiber was present in the meal. A significant proportion of fiber (notably soluble) can, in effect, substantially diminish the absorption of the said calories.
- Studies by L. Fakambi on fermented cheeses showed that if they are rich in calcium (Swiss), the calcium in the cheese retains a part of the fats that are not absorbed by the body. The corresponding calories then end up in the stool.
- The "nature" of calories also influences what happens to them in the body. Saturated fats, for example, are easily stored, while polyunsaturated fats (notably omega 3) are more readily used and, therefore, burned.
- Several studies (J. LeBlanc, etc.) have shown that levels of caloric expenditure due to food digestion (thermogenesis) differ greatly according to whether we eat the same number of calories in one single meal or in four to six spaced out meals. The more the meals are broken up, the greater the caloric expenditure.
- Finally, the simple calculation of calories does not take into consideration the time of day nutrients are absorbed. It has been shown that the absorption of carbohydrates, fats, and proteins varies according to different hours of the day and even according to the seasons (chronobiology). Their absorption also depends on

the chemical environment that nutrients encounter when they reach the small intestine. The chemical environment depends on the kinds of nutrients, the order of their arrival, and their volume.

That's why any calculation of calories that doesn't take all of these additional factors into account borders on the absurd.

How many of you have been victims of this unfounded theory of energy balance, which has tried to convince us that the human body functions like a common furnace?

You have most likely come across overweight people in your group of friends who have tried starving themselves in order to lose weight. This is especially true among women. Psychiatrists' offices are filled with women for whom nervous depression comes from the application of the calorie theory. Upon entering the infernal cycle, these women rapidly become enslaved by it because they know that stopping will lead back to a weight gain even greater that the one with which they began.

Most members of the medical world completely hide from this subject. They know well that their patients aren't losing weight, but they suspect the patients of not following the rules of the game and of sneaking food in secret. Certain pseudo-professionals in the nutrition field have even organized group therapy sessions during which overweight people confess either their weight loss, welcomed with applause, or their weight gain, received with boos and hisses. Such practices embody ridicule and mental cruelty.

Moreover, prescribing a 1400-calorie diet without specifying which foods to eat, as do many traditional dieticians, is not sufficient. It all comes back to only focusing on the pure energy aspect of food without considering its nutritional value. Those in the medical field (save certain specialists) won't even question their basic understanding of nutritional value in this domain. When it comes to nutrition, though, except for a few common points, their scientific culture is pretty slim.

Moreover, nutrition is not an area that particularly interests doctors. I came to realize that among the doctors whom I am working with, most came to be interested in nutrition and in doing the research because they, themselves, had a serious weight problem that they wanted to resolve. The upsetting, even scandalous thing is that we allowed the idea that the calorie theory had a real scientific foundation to develop into a generally accepted rule. This theory unfortunately acquired its status of nobility and has now become one of the principal cultural givens of our western civilization.

The calorie theory has reached such a point that there is not a restaurant chain, a neighborhood diner, or even a military canteen that does not post the number of calories in each of their meals. Not a single week goes by that a number of women's magazines do not feature weight loss on their front page. They let us in on the latest menus put together by a team of professional dieticians who, in light of the calorie theory, offer you something like, "an orange for breakfast, half a piece of toast at 11:00, a chick pea at noon and an olive in the evening..."

Remember that it is always professional dieticians who make the pitch.

In his book *La cuisine du bien maigrir* (published by Odile Jacob), Dr. Jacques Fricker, a well known nutritionist in France, suggests low-calorie recipes "calculated to the slightest calorie" – crab meat: 199 calories (and not 200 or 201), sautéed veal milanaise: 299 calories (and not 300), poires souflées: 156 calories. Not one more, not one less. It is absurd to pay so much attention to such a variable subject.

We can nonetheless ask ourselves why the calorie-cutting approach was able to fool us for such a long time. There are two responses to this question. The first is that a low-calorie diet often produces results. Food deprivation, on which the diet is founded, has to lead to a certain loss of weight. But, as we have already seen, this result does not last. Not only will the dieter inevitably go back to his or her original weight, but also he or she will most likely surpass it.

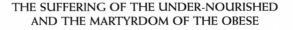

THE SUFFERING OF THE UNDER-NOURISHED
AND THE MARTYRDOM OF THE OBESE

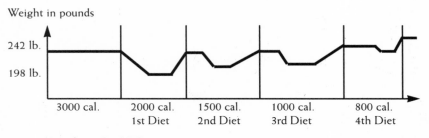

According to Dr. J.P. Ruasse:

This curve shows that following successive low-calorie diets leads to a resistance to weight loss and can even cause actual obesity.

Thus, we see that the more we lower caloric intake, the less effective the diet, and the more the body tends not only to gain back its original weight, but also to make up supplementary fat reserves.

The second reason is that "low-calorie" has these days become a big business. The term has become such an economic issue that we now face a virtual lobby of which the food industry and a few lost chefs, with the help of degreed dieticians, are now the principle beneficiaries.

The calorie theory is false, and now you know why. But that doesn't mean that you are rid of it because, at this point, it is so firmly embedded in your mind that you will continue to find yourself thinking along those lines for a long time. When we get to the eating Method that I recommend in this book, it will very possibly bother you, in that what I suggest may appear to be in total contradiction with this famous theory. If that's the case, reread this chapter until things become perfectly clear for you.

Chapter 2

THE DIFFERENT TYPES OF FOOD

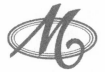

If you want to succeed at creating a veritable management of your diet, which is the key to the mastering of your weight, the first step in your training will consist of learning to recognize the foods that are commonly available to you.

Just the same, you must be made aware that the present chapter necessarily is of a technical nature. But remember, it is possible for everyone to master it.

Once you take on the learning of any discipline (sports, for example), you must first surmount a necessary step which consists of assimilating the basic technology. It is from there that you will be able to make serious progress with what follows.

Some of the information you will be given in this chapter will seem *à priori* already familiar, and you may be tempted to pass by some of the reading.

On the contrary, double your attention to it because you have been told so many erroneous things in the domain of nutrition that it is better for you to be suspicious.

Foods are edible substances that contain a certain number of nutrients such as proteins, fats, carbohydrates, vitamins, minerals and trace elements. They also contain water and non-digestible materials, like fiber.

PROTEINS (or PROTIDS)

These are the organic cells that make up living matter: muscles, organs, the liver, the brain, the skeletal structure, etc. They are made of simpler molecules called amino acids. Some amino acids are produced by the body, but mostly they are introduced into the system through different ingested foods.

Protein comes from two sources:

Animal sources: meats, fish, cheese, eggs, and dairy products.

Vegetable sources: soy, almonds, hazelnuts, whole grains, and certain legumes (like beans and lentils).

The ideal would be to consume as many proteins from vegetable sources as from animal sources. But that is not always easy to do.

Proteins are indispensable to the body:

-for the construction of cellular structures as an eventual source of energy, after their transformation into glucose (the Krebs cycle),

-to make certain hormones and neurotransmitters.[1]

-for building up nucleic acids (necessary for reproduction).

A diet deficient in proteins can lead to serious bodily consequences: muscle breakdown, immune deficiency, wrinkling of the skin, etc. Daily protein intake must be around sixty grams per day for children and ninety grams for adolescents. Adults

---

[1] Neurotransmitter: chemical substance released by nerve endings, under the influence of a stimulus and producing an adapted biological effect.

must consume one gram of protein per kg (2.2 lb.) of body weight per day, with a minimum of 55 grams per day for women and 70 grams per day for men. In addition, for adults, proteins must account for at least 15% of their daily energy intake.

But protein intake can, without disadvantages, be greater (1.2 to 1.5 grams of protein per kg (or 2.2 lb.) per day) provided enough fluids are drunk to eliminate the waste from protein metabolism (uric acid, urea, lactic acid). Greater protein intake can effectively help in your weight loss phase. First, because its metabolism leads to greater energy expenditure than other foods. But also because it causes you to feel fuller more quickly. According to Professor D. Tomé, "It seems that an adult's regulatory capacity allows him or her to adapt to a wide range of protein intake, between 0.6 and 2 grams per kg (2.2 lb.) per day, without major visible repercussions on overall health" (Chole-doc.no45, Jan/Feb.98).

Except for eggs, animal or vegetable proteins alone do not provide the necessary balance of amino acids. The absence of one amino acid can limit absorption of other amino acids. Your diet must therefore associate proteins of both animal and vegetable origin.

A diet based solely on vegetable proteins (vegetarianism) would be unbalanced. It would notably lack cysteine, causing problems in the hair and nails. On the other hand, a vegetarian diet including eggs and dairy products can be completely balanced.

CARBOHYDRATES

Carbohydrates are molecules made up of carbon, oxygen, and hydrogen. They are metabolized into glucose, which is a major energy source for the body, especially because it is readily useable. We can distinguish several types of carbohydrates based on the complexity of their molecules.

Carbohydrate classification:
- Carbohydrates made up of a single molecule (simple sugars):
- <u>glucose</u>, found in honey and fruit
- <u>fructose</u>, also found in honey and fruit
- <u>galactose</u>, from milk

- Carbohydrates made up of two molecules (double sugars):
- <u>saccharide</u> (white sugar extracted from beets or sugar cane) made up of glucose and fructose
- <u>lactose</u> (glucose and galactose) the glucose from the milk of mammals
- <u>maltose</u> (glucose and glucose) the main sugar found in beer, also found in corn

- Carbohydrates made up of several molecules (complex sugars):
- <u>starch</u>, whose molecules contain hundreds of glucose molecules, which are also found in:
- <u>grains</u>: wheat, corn, rice
- <u>tubers</u>: potatoes, yams, artichokes
- <u>roots</u>: rutabaga
- <u>grains or legumes</u>: beans, lentils, peas, chickpeas, snow peas, soy beans

The classification into slow and quick sugars is wrong!

For a long time we placed carbohydrates into two distinct categories, based on how long we thought it took the body to absorb them: quick sugars and slow sugars. Under the heading "quick sugars" were the simple sugars and double sugars like glucose and saccharide, found in refined sugar (from sugar cane or sugar beets), honey, and fruit.

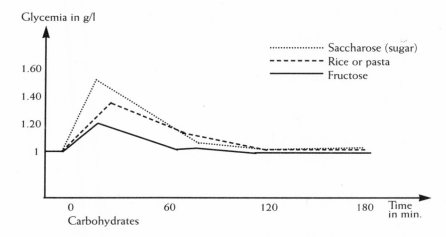

The term "quick sugars" was based on the belief that because of the simplicity of the carbohydrate molecules, they were rapidly absorbed by the body soon after ingestion. Inversely, we placed under the category of "slow sugars" all carbohydrates made up of complex molecules, which had to be chemically transformed into simple sugars (glucose) during digestion. This was notably true of starches, where glucose was released – so we thought – slowly and progressively into the body.

Today, this classification is completely <u>outdated</u>, because it is based on erroneous thinking. Recent experiments have proven that, in effect, the complexity of the carbohydrate molecule does not determine the speed at which glucose is released and used by the body. The glycemic peak, meaning the maximal absorption level, of all carbohydrates, eaten alone on an empty stomach, occurs in the same amount of time (around half an hour after their ingestion).

Instead of discussing assimilation speed, it would make more sense to study carbohydrates based on the rise in glycemia that they cause, that is, the quantity of glucose they cause the body to produce. Therefore, all scientists (cf. bibliography) have admitted that the classification of carbohydrates must be done based on their hyperglycemic potential, defined by the concept of the glycemic index. But in order to help you to understand the meaning of the glycemic index, which is one of the main foundations of the Montignac Method, we should first discuss the essential notion of glycemia.

What is glycemia?

First, remember that carbohydrates are an important source of fuel for the body. They are indispensable to the functioning of the brain. That is why they are constantly present in the blood. This presence is identified by what we will call the glycemia level, which, on an empty stomach, is "normally" about one gram of carbohydrates (sugar) per liter (approx. 1 quart) of blood. If the level goes below this norm, the secretion of a pancreatic hormone, glucagon, reestablishes the normal level. When we eat a carbohydrate, the absorption of corresponding glucose will cause a rise in glycemia.

At first, glycemia will increase (more or less according to the type of carbohydrate ingested) until it reaches a maximum, which we call the glycemic peak. The pancreas (a major organ in the regulation of metabolic processes) will then secrete another hormone insulin, the objective being to eliminate the excess

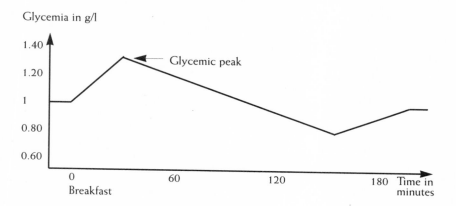

Glycemia in g/l

glucose in the blood and to store it elsewhere in the body (the liver and muscles) in case it is needed. Under the effect of the insulin, the glycemia level becomes lower until finally going back to normal.

The glycemic index

The glycemic potential of each carbohydrate is defined by its glycemic ability and is measured by the glycemic index, first established in 1976. It corresponds to the measure of the triangular surface of the hyperglycemic curve induced by carbohydrate ingestion. We arbitrarily give glucose an index of 100, which represents the triangular surface of the corresponding hyperglycemic curve. The glycemic index of other carbohydrates, therefore, is calculated by the following formula:

$$\frac{\text{Triangular surface of tested carbohydrate}}{\text{Triangular surface of glucose}} \times 100$$

The glycemic index rises according to the level of hyperglycemia. Thus, the higher the glycemic index, the higher the hyperglycemia induced by the carbohydrate will be.

It should be noted that industrial processing and methods of preparing and cooking carbohydrates can raise their glycemic

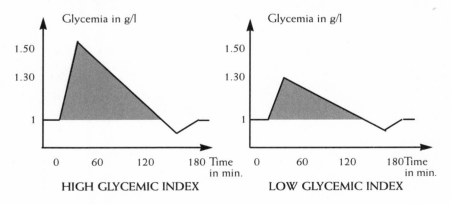

HIGH GLYCEMIC INDEX   LOW GLYCEMIC INDEX

39

index (corn flakes 85, corn 70, instant potatoes 95, boiled potatoes 70). We also know that it is not only the composition of starch (ratio of amylase to amylopectin), but also the amount of protein and fiber, and the quality of fiber in carbohydrate-rich foods, that cause their indexes to be either low or high (hamburger rolls 85, white bread, baguette 70, whole wheat bread 40, white rice 70, and brown rice 50).

In order to simplify matters, I propose dividing carbohydrates into two categories: "good carbohydrates" (having a low glycemic index) and "bad carbohydrates" (having a high glycemic index). In the following chapters this distinction will show you, among other things, the reasons why you are overweight.

Bad carbohydrates

These are the carbohydrates whose assimilation causes a significant rise in glucose in the blood (hyperglycemia). This is true of all forms of table sugar (either pure or in other foods, such as pastries), but it is also true of all industrially refined carbohydrates, like white flour, white rice, corn, as well as potatoes.

Good carbohydrates

Unlike bad carbohydrates, these are not markedly assimilated by the body, resulting in less of a rise in blood sugar (glycemia). This is true of unrefined flours, brown rice, and particularly certain starchy foods, like lentils and kidney beans. It is especially true of most fruits and all vegetables that contain fiber (cabbage, broccoli, cauliflower, lettuce, green beans, leeks, etc.)

LIPIDS (or FATS)

Lipids are complex molecules, more commonly known as fatty acids. We distinguish, according to their origin, two main lipid categories:

GLYCEMIC INDEX CHART

High Glycemic Index Carbohydrates		Low Glycemic Index Carbohydrates	
Maltose (beer)	110	Whole wheat or bran bread	50
Glucose	100	Brown rice	50
Baked potatoes	95	Basmati rice	50
French fries	95	Canned peas	50
Rice flour	95	Sweet potatoes	50
Modified starch	95	Whole wheat pasta	50
Mashed potatoes	90	Spaghetti (al dente)	45
Potato chips	90	Fresh peas	40
Honey	85	Whole wheat, sugar-free	
Hamburger rolls	85	cereal	40
Cooked carrots	85	Oatmeal	40
Corn flakes, popcorn	85	Whole grain pasta	40
Instant rice	85	Kidney beans	40
Rice cakes	85	Fresh unsweetened fruit juice	40
Puffed rice	85	Pumpernickel bread	40
Cooked broad beans	80	Rye bread	40
Pumpkin	75	100% integral bread	40
Watermelon	75	Figs, dried apricots	35
Sugar (saccharose)	70	Genuine indian corn	35
White bread		Wild rice	35
(baguette)	70	Quinoa	35
Refined sweetened		Raw carrots	30
cereals	70	Dairy products	30
Chocolate bars	70	Dried beans	30
Boiled peeled potatoes	70	Brown or yellow lentils	30
Cola, soda	70	Chickpeas	30
Cookies	70	Fresh fruit	30
Corn	70	Green beans	30
White rice	70	Soy vermicelli	30
Noodles, ravioli	70	Sugar-free marmalade	22
Raisins	65	Green lentils	22
Boiled unpeeled		Split peas	22
potatoes	65	Dark chocolate (>70% cacao)	22
Beets	65	Fructose	20
Sweetened preserves	65	Soy, peanuts	15
Refined semolina	60	Fresh apricots	15
Long-grain rice	60	Green vegetables, tomatoes,	
Bananas, cantaloupe	60	eggplant, zucchini, garlic,	
Well-cooked white		onions, etc.	<15
spaghetti	55		
Shortbread cookies	55		

- *ANIMAL LIPIDS*, contained in meat, fish, butter, eggs, cheese, sour cream, etc.
- *VEGETABLE LIPIDS*, are peanut oil, olive oil, nut oils, margarine, etc.

We can also classify lipids into three categories according to the nature of their fatty acids:

- *SATURATED FATS*, found in meat, eggs, and whole-fat dairy products (milk, butter, cream, cheese)
- *MONOUNSATURATED FATS*, found mostly in olive oil, fats from goose and duck, liver paté;
- *POLYUNSATURATED VEGETABLE FATS*: oil from seeds (mainly sunflower) and oleaginous fruits. Margarine is made by hydrogenating a polyunsaturated fat.
- *POLYUNSATURATED ANIMAL FATS*, found mostly in fish, but also in shellfish.

Lipids are necessary to any diet. They provide storable energy that is readily available according to the body's needs. They control the formation of membranes and cells and contribute to the composition of tissues, especially those of the nervous system. Later, you will see the importance of making the distinction between good and bad fats.

What's more, fatty foods contain a number of vitamins (A, D, E, and K) and essential fats (linoleic acid and linolenic acid) and aid in the development of various hormones. Generally, we eat too much bad fat. Fried foods, donuts, useless sauces, and foods cooked with grease have invaded our diets, even though we could easily enjoy a lighter cuisine that is just as delicious, without overindulging.

Certain lipids are responsible for a rise in cholesterol, but there are actually two types of cholesterol: "good" and "bad". The objective is to maintain a normal total cholesterol level, keeping the level of good cholesterol (HDL cholesterol) as high as possible and the level of bad cholesterol (LDL cholesterol) as low as possible. Not all lipids cause an increase in "bad" cholesterol; on the contrary, some even tend to significantly lower it. In fact, to be totally objective, fats should be classified into three categories:

FATS THAT RAISE CHOLESTEROL:
These are saturated fats found in meat, cold cuts, butter, cheese, lard, whole dairy products, and palm oil.

FATS THAT ONLY SLIGHTLY AFFECT CHOLESTEROL:
These are found in shellfish, eggs, and skinless poultry.

FATS THAT LOWER CHOLESTEROL:
These are vegetable oils: olive, rapeseed, sunflower, corn, etc.

Fish fats do not really affect the metabolism of cholesterol but prevent cardiovascular diseases by reducing triglycerides and hindering blood clots. It is thus necessary to eat fatty fish (salmon, tuna, mackerel, herring, and sardines).

The Method of weight loss I offer you in this book is essentially based on choosing between "good" and "bad" carbohydrates. If you have high cholesterol, you will be encouraged to choose between "good" and "bad" fats in order to prevent the risk of cardiovascular diseases[2] for good.

DIETARY FIBER

Dietary fibers are particularly contained in carbohydrates with a low glycemic index: vegetables, legumes, fruit, and unrefined grains. They are also found in foods said to be unprocessed. Even

---

[2] An entire chapter is devoted to hypercholesterolemia, as well as to its cardiovascular risks; see Chapter 8.

though it has basically no energetic value, dietary fiber plays an extremely important role in digestion. They especially reduce the absorption of carbohydrates, thus causing a lower glycemia.

There are two kinds of fiber:

Insoluble fiber (cellulose, hemicellulose) provides good intestinal transit. Its absence (or at least deficiency) is the cause of most cases of constipation.

Soluble fiber (gum, pectin) limits digestive absorption, especially of lipids, and lowers the risk of atherosclerosis.

Fiber-rich foods are also rich in vitamins, trace elements[3] and mineral salts. Insufficient amounts of these can cause serious deficiencies. Fiber can also limit the toxic effects of certain chemical substances, such as additives and colorants. According to gastroenterologists, certain kinds of fiber can protect the colon

SOURCES OF FIBER
and their concentrations for a 3.5-ounce serving

Grains		Legumes		Dried oleaginous fruits	
Bran	40g	Dried beans	25g	Dried coconut	24g
Multi-grain bread	13g	Split peas	23g	Dried figs	18g
Whole wheat flour	9g	Lentils	12g	Almonds	14g
Brown rice	5g	Chickpeas	2g	Raisins	7g
White rice	1g			Dates	9g
White bread	2.5g			Peanuts	8g
Green vegetables		Cabbage	4g	Fresh fruits	
Cooked peas	12g	Radishes	3g	Raspberries	8g
Parsley	19g	Mushrooms	2.5g	Pears in skin	3g
Cooked spinach	7g	Carrots	2g	Apples in skin	3g
Romaine	5g	Lettuce	2g	Strawberries	3g
Artichokes	4g			Peaches	2g
Leeks	4g				

---

[3] Trace elements: metals or metalloids present in infinitesimal amounts in the human body, which are necessary as catalysts for certain chemical reactions in the body.

and rectum from a number of risks, especially cancers of the digestive system.

For the past few decades, changes in lifestyle of industrialized countries have led to a significant decrease in fiber consumption. The French currently consume less than 20g of fiber per day (Americans less than 10g) even though the recommended amount is between 30 and 40g. In 1925, the French consumed 7.3 kg (about 16 lbs.) of dried beans (particularly rich in fiber) per inhabitant per year. Today they consume no more than 1.3 kg (less than 3 lbs.); that is, 5.6 times less. The basis of the Italian diet has always been pasta. Thirty years ago, Italians essentially ate vegetables (rich in fiber) and whole-wheat pasta; that is, made with unrefined flour containing wheat fiber.

Today with the changes in lifestyle, meat has replaced legumes and vegetables. Also, pasta is made with refined white flour, meaning that the fiber has been taken out of it. Medical authorities of this country now attribute the rise in obesity and the alarming proliferation of digestive cancers to this situation.[4]

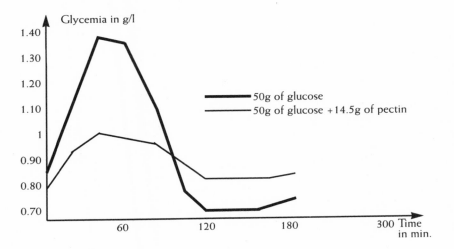

----

[4] See the publications of Pr. Giacosa, chief of service Nutrition of the National Center of Research on Gene Cancer.

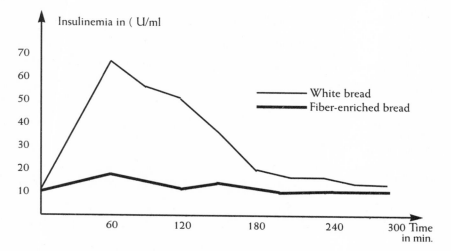

It has been shown that fiber has an indirect beneficial effect on obesity. Its introduction into the diet can lower glycemia as well as insulinemia, (the level of insulin in the blood), which is, as we will see in the following chapter, responsible for the storage of excess fats. The diagrams below show that the presence of fiber in consumed carbohydrates with a high glycemic index leads to a reduction in glycemia and insulinemia.

SUMMARY

PROTEINS are substances found in many foods of animal and vegetable origin. They are found in meat, fish, eggs, dairy products (even skim), legumes, unrefined foods and certain soy products. They are necessary for the body and do not cause weight gain.

CARBOHYDRATES are substances that are metabolized into glucose. They are found in sweet foods (fruit, honey) and starchy foods (legumes, flour, roots, tubers, and grains). All carbohydrates are absorbed (when ingested on an empty stomach) in the same amount of time. This is why the old classification of carbohydrates into "slow" sugars and "quick" sugars is erroneous. They should be classified based on their glycemic potential, measured by the glycemic index. We can therefore make the distinction between "good carbohydrates" having a low glycemic index, and "bad carbohydrates" having a high glycemic index.

LIPIDS come from both plants and animals. They are fatty acids found in meat, fish, dairy products, and oils (olive, sunflower, walnut, etc.). Some fatty acids cause a rise in cholesterol (meat, whole milk products, palm oil) while others lower cholesterol (olive oil, fruits, fish fats, and chocolate).

FIBER is a non-energy producing substance contained in foods having a low glycemic index, like green vegetables (lettuce, endives, leeks, spinach, green beans, etc.) and certain dried beans, fruits, and whole grains. Fiber-rich foods should be consumed in large quantities because of their nutritional interest and their contribution to weight loss.

CHAPTER 2

Chapter 3

WHERE DO THE EXTRA POUNDS COME FROM?

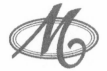

In Chapter 1 we saw what was wrong with the traditional idea that calories are responsible for weight gain. Nutritionists and other dieticians thought that the human body functioned as a simple furnace with, on one hand, the calories gained by eating, and on the other hand, the calories burned by the functioning of the human body. Therefore, we thought for a long time that if some people were overweight, it was because they ate too much or they did not do enough physical exercise.

In this chapter you will learn why this hypothesis is false. More importantly, you will come to understand that extra pounds are essentially the result of abnormally stored energy from certain metabolic mechanisms put in place by poor choices of food. Thus, you will realize that it is the qualitative factor of foods more so than their quantitative factor that dictates weight gain. People gain weight then, not necessarily because they eat too much, but because they eat poorly.

THE ROAD TO HYPERINSULINISM

Since 1979, nutrition researchers have clearly demonstrated the technical (metabolic) process behind weight gain. All concluded that "hyperinsulinism is present in all cases of obesity, no matter what the species or mechanism."[5] And all the studies show that this hyperinsulinism is proportional to the magnitude of excess weight. It has a greater effect on androgynous obesity (situated above the belt) than on gynecoid obesity (in the bottom half of the body).

This means that someone who is only ten to twenty pounds overweight has moderately hyperinsulinism, and that someone who is obese has <u>highly hyperinsulinism</u>. We can logically conclude, then, that the real difference between a thin and a fat person is that the fat person produces high levels of insulin and that the thin person does not.

Let us imagine that two people live together and eat exactly the same thing (and the same number of calories) every day. If after several years, one is fat and the other is not, there is not a single good explanation, except that the one who is fat suffers from hyperinsulinism and the other does not. To understand hyperinsulinism, we must first talk about insulin.

In the last chapter you learned the definition of glycemia: the level of glucose (sugar) in the blood. As specified, the normal level of glycemia on an empty stomach is around one gram per two pints of blood. We also saw that as this level lowers (hypoglycemia), an important organ in the regulation of metabolic processes, the pancreas, secretes a hormone called glucagon, whose role is to release a new supply of glucose into the blood. Glucagon, therefore, raises the level of glycemia.

---

[5] Jeanrenaud B. (Insulin and obesity, Diabetologia 1979, 17, 133-138)

But when the level of glycemia goes up (hyperglycemia), which happens after having eaten a meal, especially a meal containing carbohydrates, the pancreas secretes another hormone, insulin, whose role is to <u>lower glycemia</u>. So the amount of insulin needed to bring glycemia back to normal is proportional to the level of glycemia present. In other words, if glycemia is low, the secretion of insulin will be low. If glycemia is very high, the secretion of insulin will be high.

This is exactly what happens in a thin person. The amount of insulin secreted by the pancreas is always exactly proportional to the level of glycemia. On the other hand, for those who are overweight and especially for obese people, things happen differently.

As soon as the glycemic peak is attained, the pancreas begins to secrete insulin, but instead of releasing it into the blood in the exact quantity necessary to bring glycemia to its normal level, it will secrete <u>way too much</u>. Thus, to have hyperinsulinism is to have a pancreas that secretes an amount of insulin that does not correspond to the level of glycemia present. And if hyperinsulinism is responsible for weight gain, it also puts metabolic mechanisms in place (lipogenesis) that abnormally cause the body to abnormally store some of the fats consumed during the last meal.

In the absence of hyperinsulinism, these trapped and stored fats would have undergone another metabolic process that would have oxidized them, allowing them to be used beneficially by the body. This is why we say that a thin person "burns" all the calories he or she consumes, especially fat calories. On the other hand, an obese person has a greater propensity to store fats than a thin person because of hyperinsulinism and also a possible insulinoresistance[7] (see footnote on next page).

Thus hyperinsulinism is, if not a disease, at least a problem with metabolism. The overweight and obese are individuals whose pancreases are more or less dysfunctional. When this was discovered at the beginning of the 1980s, researchers thought (and most still think) that if someone was hyperinsulinic it was the fault of "bad luck", that is, that they blamed heredity. Because those same researchers had noticed that hyperinsulinism went away with the pounds, the only concrete advice they gave to overweight or obese people was to lose weight.

What is more, this is what made most people believe that hyperinsulinism was the consequence of being overweight and of obesity, which were the result of excessive consumption and insufficient use of calories. The conclusion for all of these "specialists" was simple (or better yet simplistic): "the only way to get rid of hyperinsulinism is to lose weight, and to lose weight one must reduce the overall intake of calories and increase physical activity."[8] Following this, a narrow, Manechaen view of hyperinsulinism will not lead us much further.

THE OTHER HYPOTHESIS

By way of the discoveries I had made with diabetes researchers on this new classification of carbohydrates based on their

---

[7]A *worsening* factor: *insulinoresistance*. For the obese person, hyperinsulinism is worsened by the phenomenon of *insulinoresistance*. In reaction to hyperglycemia, the pancreas secretes, as we saw, a large amount of insulin. Then, this quantity of insulin, not only excessive, but also poorly recognized by the body, without a doubt because the sensitivity of the receptors is defective. As hyperglycemia persists abnormally, the pancreas has a tendency to get out of control and then secrete a new dose of insulin, which only worsens the hyperinulism. It therefore creates a vicious circle for itself, in which hyperinsulinism supports *insulinoresistance*. Outside of the consequence that we know on the storing of fats, there is also, because of insulinoresistance, a supplementary risk of a reactionary hypoglycemia.

[8] Dr. Jacques Fricker – La métabolisme de l'obésité – *La recherche* 1989, 20, 207, 200-208

glycemic index, I was attacking the problem from a different angle. Contrary to those who had concluded that hyperinsulinism was caused by obesity, I formulated the hypothesis that obesity was caused by hyperinsulinism. In other words, <u>hyperinsulinism was the cause and not the consequence of weight gain</u>.

It was thus appropriate to make the following observation:

If, as I had observed, consuming carbohydrates with a low glycemic index stopped weight gain (and even triggered weight loss) it must be that it diminished (even stopped) its cause: hyperinsulinism.

The hypothesis that could be made from this observation was the following:

Obesity can only be the consequence of hyperinsulinism. But hyperinsulinism is, itself, the consequence of high hyperglycemia. And high hyperglycemia is, itself, the consequence of an excessive consumption of carbohydrates with a high glycemic index. In other words, the consumption of carbohydrates with a high glycemic index is indirectly (via hyperglycemia and hyperinsulinism) responsible for weight gain by favoring the storage of lipids as well as excess glucose, which is transformed into fat. Hyperinsulinism, in some ways, is the "catalyst" of obesity.

To ward off (even stop) weight gain, it is sufficient to combat the initial cause, that is, to change eating habits by adopting a diet where carbohydrates are exclusively chosen among those having a low glycemic index.

THE RESULTANT GLYCEMIA OF THE MEAL

Since the 1980s, a large number of studies on diabetes have been done on glycemic indexes. Today, these studies provide us with a good understanding of the different metabolic phenomena caused by our choices of carbohydrates. Particularly, we know that the glycemic index of a carbohydrate can vary based on several parameters:

- The specific variety: certain varieties of rice for example (especially Basmati), can have a low index (50) while others (sticky rice) can have a high one (70).

- The method of cooking: raw carrots have a low index (35) while the index of cooked carrots is 85. Potatoes' indexes grow according to the way in which they are cooked: 65 if they are cooked unpeeled in water, 70 if they are peeled before cooking, 90 if they are mashed, and 95 if they are baked or fried.

- Industrial treatment or processing: regular corn has an index of 70, but it goes up to 85 when made into corn flakes or popcorn. White pasta made under high extrusion pressure, like spaghetti, has a low glycemic index (40 to 45 depending on the cooking), while ravioli and macaroni, which are not extruded, have a high index (70).

- The fiber and protein content: lentils, which contain fiber (especially soluble) and protein have a very low glycemic index (22 to 30) compared to other starchy foods such as potatoes. In the same way, soy, which contains a high level of protein, has a very low glycemic index.

Meals are generally complex in the sense that they are usually made up of various foods. Some foods can raise the level of glycemia, others, on the other hand, help to moderate it. The important factor is the resulting glycemia of the meal. This is what will determine the final level of hyperglycemia and indirectly (if it is high) hyperinsulinism, which is responsible for the abnormal storage of fats.

OUR SOCIETY'S DIETARY TRENDS

In the preceding paragraphs we saw that the original cause of weight gain is the ingestion of carbohydrates containing a high glycemic index, which causes abnormal storage of fats. But we can legitimately ask ourselves how some people who eat carbohydrates with high glycemic indexes every day can stay ideally thin. The response is simple. It is because their pancreas, which is (still) in good shape, again does not yet suffer from hyperinsulinism.

But can a person stay thin all his or her life while continuing to eat a hyperglycemic diet? In effect, it is possible but less and less probable. You will see why.

Some people can, in effect, stay thin their whole life even though they have poor eating habits. This means that when they were born they had a pancreas in very good shape and, despite high hyperglycemia, which they induced all their life by eating bad carbohydrates, their pancreas was resistant enough to not allow hyperinsulinism to set in.

Other people (most people) also started out with a healthy pancreas that allowed them to stay thin for many years despite their poor eating habits. Then, around the age of 30 or 35, and especially after 40, they begin to gain weight. Some even become obese and diabetic in their late years. This means that their pancreas resisted during several decades but that, because of the stress put on it day after day, year after year, to fight against permanent hyperglycemia, it finally "gave in." A little like a motor, which little by little, because of the poor treatment it receives, works more and more poorly.

And then there are those (like me) who were born with an already unhealthy pancreas. This is why we logically attribute this deficiency to heredity. It is true that when one has obese parents (whose bodies produce too much insulin) there is a strong probability that his or her own pancreas will be fragile. It is practically sure, in any case, if the dietary habits developed at a young age are highly hyperglycemic.

In 1997 the World Health Organization denounced the world's obesity epidemic. Until that time, we thought that only Americans had a problem with obesity. We then realized that this was a general problem in the western countries. Yet the most surprising thing is that all the countries on the planet have since been touched by what could be considered actual contamination.

Also in 1997, a large study showed that in the United States[9] obesity, paradoxically, has increased by 31% over the last 10 years, even though during the same period the average caloric intake had decreased, the consumption of fats had fallen by 11%, and the number of people consuming low fat products had gone from 19% to 76%. This survey showed that the cause of weight gain was independent of the quantity of calories taken in, since that quantity had even significantly decreased. It would therefore tend to confirm that, rather, the degradation of the modern diet's nutritional quality has caused this situation.

Looking closely at the glycemic index table (p.41), we see that the foods in the left-hand column, meaning those having a high glycemic index, are foods that are refined (flour, sugar, white rice), processed (corn flakes, puffed rice, modified starches, chocolate bars), or "new" foods that have only been eaten regularly for fewer than two centuries (potatoes, white flour, or, again, sugar). It is not difficult to see that all of these foods are precisely those consumed today in most Western countries and

---

[9] Adrian F. *Divergent trends in Obesity and fat intake pattern* "The American paradox" Am.J.Med. 1997; 102: 259-264)

that, with worldwide spread, they are invading the eating habits of the rest of the world.

Inversely, we should note that the carbohydrates listed in the right-hand column of the table, meaning those with a low glycemic index, correspond, for the most part, to foods that we no longer eat (whole wheat bread, whole grains, unrefined flour, brown rice, etc.), foods that are rarely eaten (lentils, dried beans, split peas, chickpeas, etc.), or else foods that are not eaten frequently enough (fruits, green vegetable, etc.) These are all foods that were eaten mainly in the past, even just 50 years ago.

The diet of the past (just several decades ago) was primarily composed of only <u>slightly glycemic</u> foods, that is, whose glycemic index was low. Because the resulting glycemia of the meal was low, our ancestors' pancreases were not frequently needed for their insulinic function, therefore, the risk of hyperinsulinism was low.

This is also what explains the fact that there were very few obese people in Western countries at the beginning of the 20th century (fewer than 3% compared to 20%-33% today) and that only 10%-20% of the population had a slight weight problem compared to 30% to 65% today, depending on the country. Inversely, our modern eating habits favor foods with a high glycemic index. Thus, the resulting glycemia of our contemporary meals is particularly high, excessively stimulating the pancreas and progressively leading to a hypersecretion of insulin: hyperinsulinism.

Although eating habits remained constant for millenniums, the Western diet has been changing since the beginning of the 20th century. In effect, we have progressively moved from a low glycemic diet mode to a very hyperglycemic one. Because of this increasingly hyperglycemic diet, our contemporaries' pancreases have been increasingly needed. The most sensitive pancreases have quickly "given up" causing hyperinsulinism. The number of people able to resist has become lower and lower, which means that the population of overweight and obese people continues to grow.

According to a prospective study done in 1997, 100% of Americans should be obese in 2039 if the trends of these last thirty years continue into the years to come.

THE AMERICAN DIETARY MODEL

We already mentioned that obesity is unfortunately worse in the United States than anywhere else in the world – three times worse than in France. So let us look at the main components of the American diet and, in particular, those involving fast food, which represent their essential eating habits.

Americans mainly consume:

- Refined white flour (index 85) found in hamburger and hotdog rolls, sandwich bread, cookies, and crackers.

- Sugar (index 70) found in industrial products (canned foods, mustard, ketchup, crackers, cookies, ready-made meals) as well as in drinks (especially soft drinks, fruit juices, instant iced tea)

- Potatoes essentially eaten fried (index 95)

- Corn consumed unrefined (index 70) or made into corn flakes or popcorn (index 85)

- White rice mass-produced (index 70) or made into rice cakes (index 85)

Not to mention the fact that Americans drink large amounts of beer (index 110) and mainly consume pre-cooked, processed foods, which all contain corn syrup (index 100), maltodextrins (index 100) and modified starches (index 95). Thus, it is easy to deduce that there is a strict correlation between the American diet and its resulting metabolic pathologies: obesity, diabetes and even cardiovascular pathologies.

Moreover, it is interesting to note that obesity in the US is most prevalent among the lower classes of society. It is precisely among these populations that the hyperglycemic foods listed above are most often consumed. Inversely, the wealthier Americans are, the more traditionally they tend to eat, and the less they are victims of obesity.

THE END OF THE FRENCH MODEL

Even today, the French occupy the lowest point in the Western world on the average weight curve. In other words, although there are more and more overweight and obese people in France, this progression is lower than that of Anglo-Saxons.

One has only to examine the French diet to understand why. The reason is without a doubt linked to the fact that the French have better resisted, because of their strong traditions, the spread of North American eating habits. Just the same, French young people have not resisted as well as their parents. That is why the number of obese people in this category has been increasing at an alarming rate for twenty years. It is possible that in two or three generations, the French population will be as hyperinsulinic (therefore obese) as the Anglo-Saxons.

In conclusion, the answer to the title of this chapter is that it is by mainly consuming carbohydrates with a high glycemic index (associated with fat storage) that we gain extra pounds.

In the following chapter you will learn how to get rid of those pounds for good. This is the goal of the Montignac Method.

Chapter 4

THE METHOD
PHASE I: WEIGHT LOSS

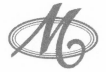

In the previous chapters, you discovered that contrary to what nutritionists believed and told us for more than half a century, the caloric content of foods is not a determining factor in weight gain. If we gain weight, and even more so if we become obese, it is not because we eat too much, but because we eat poorly.

In other words, the extra pounds are the result of poor dietary choices which set off abnormal metabolic mechanisms leading to the anomalous storage of fats.

The application of the Method will thus consist of modifying our dietary habits by recentering our choices on the foods that have a positive metabolic potential. This is essentially what we will do in Phase II, which is the crossover phase where dietary choices will permit us, above all, to avoid weight gain.

What is more, nothing is keeping you from attacking the Method by directly beginning with Phase II. The testimonies of thousands of people allow us to, in effect, affirm that you will thus be able to get rid of your extra pounds, but that can demand much more time to succeed, especially if you have a significant amount of weight to lose.

If you are impatient to get rid of your excess weight for good, then I invite you to begin by applying the principles of Phase I, which is the actual weight loss phase. It will have the advantage of correcting the dietary errors of your past and definitively putting your metabolism on the right track.

The first thing to do when beginning a project, which is moreover an ambitious project, is to fix an objective. To do this you can use the information in Chapter 12 on the calculation of your BMI.

Thus, you must determine by how much you are overweight, but know that each body is driven differently. And then, you must also keep other factors in mind: sex, age, dietary history, and heredity.

That is why it is difficult to say how many pounds you are going to be able to lose per week. For some, it will be two pounds, for others a little less. And in numerous cases, there will be a significant drop in the beginning followed by a slower loss. So do not be worried if it takes longer for you than for someone else in your entourage.

Perhaps you already have a more or less precise idea of how much you would like to lose. I know from experience that for a good number of you, if you could lose eight to ten pounds (even though you are 20 to 25 pounds overweight) you would already be happy.

I, myself, encourage you to be more demanding than that. You are undoubtedly ambitious in your personal and professional life. Be so also for your figure.

FOODS TO BE WATCHED

The fundamental principle of the Method consists of seeing to it that the resultant glycemia of your meal is the lowest possible while continuing to maintain a balanced diet and thus eating normal amounts of carbohydrates. On the other hand, these will be chosen according to their effect on glycemia. But before learning to make the right choices, let us look in detail at why it is important to be careful of certain carbohydrates.

SUGAR

This is one of the champions of the "bad carbohydrates" category. A danger sign should always accompany sugar. In effect, it is a product that can be dangerous when we eat too much of it. Unfortunately, this is the case for most of our contemporaries, especially children.

I hope to convince you of its harmful dietary role and its consequences; not only on weight gain, but also and especially on fatigue (see the chapter on glycemia), diabetes, dental cavities, and coronary diseases. Perhaps some of you are thinking that sugar is indispensable. Well no, it is not. The proof is that for tens of thousands of years, humans did not have sugar at their disposal, and they did not do too badly. In fact, they did quite well. Less than two centuries ago sugar was still a luxury that was not very accessible to the majority of the population. Today it possibly wreaks more havoc than alcohol and drugs combined, even counting their over-consumption.

But then, you ask yourself, if I cut out sugar completely, how will I be able to maintain the necessary minimum in my blood? Good question.

Know that the body needs glucose (which is a source of energy), and not sugar. Fruit, unrefined foods, legumes, and grains provide glucose. In the temporary absence of carbohydrates (like during certain sporting events), the body knows to resort to other forms of energy, from stored fats for example. So do not eat any more sugar.

You can do one of two things: you can either completely give up sugar from the beginning - and I congratulate you - or you may have to transitionally replace sugar with an artificial sweetener.[10]

BREAD

Bread could have been the object of an entire chapter because there is much to say about it, good things about the "good bread", so rare in our era, but especially bad things about the deceiving product sold by the vast majority of bakeries and supermarkets. Regular bread, made with refined flour, is completely devoid of everything necessary for normal metabolism. Nutritionally, it contributes nothing except energy in the form of starch. Digestively, it causes more or less obvious problems because all the components that contribute to good digestion are removed during the refining process.

Moreover, the whiter the bread, the worse the carbohydrate because the whiteness is what signals major refining of the flour. Whole wheat bread[11], or actual (integral) whole grain bread, made the old way with organic, unrefined flour, is quite preferable because it is much richer in fiber. This is why its glycemic index is lower (50 for whole wheat bread, 40 for real integral-whole grain bread). It is therefore less "fattening" because it causes only a small elevation in glycemia.

---

[10] See Chapter 9 on sugar.

[11] For 3 1/2 oz. of bread, there are 90 mg of magnesium in whole wheat bread and only 25 mg in white bread.

Yet as good as it is, even that bread will be temporarily eliminated from your two main meals. First of all because its glycemic index, although low, is still too high (>35) and secondly because the more carbohydrates we have during a meal, even with a low glycemic index, the greater the risk (in Phase I) of noticeably raising insulin production. If you already consume a significant amount of another starch like chickpeas or green lentils, then it is not desirable to add bread. What is more, for bread to have a glycemic index of 40 it must be made with 100% unrefined flour (without any bleaching) and its texture must be course (large grains), which you will never be sure of unless the manufacturer can guarantee it.

On the other hand, you will be able to eat bread for breakfast (it is even recommended). We will discuss this in more detail later.

STARCHES

Starches are complex carbohydrates. Some, like lentils or peas, induce a weak glycemia and are, therefore, "good carbohydrates". On the other hand, others, like potatoes, are carbohydrates with high glycemic indexes. This is why it will be necessary to eliminate them in Phase 1.

POTATOES

Here is a little history. When the potato was brought from the New World in 1540 by explorers, the French deliberately rejected this root, deeming it only good enough for pigs. They found it so bad that they refused to eat it, which was not the case in Nordic, German, Scandinavian, and Irish countries, which adopted it more willingly. It should be said that they did not really have a choice, often not having anything else to eat.

The French treated this "tuber for pigs" with contempt for more than two centuries. It was not until 1789 with a publication by Parmentier called **Treatise on the Culture and Use of the Potato** that the French decided to eat the tuber in question. The famine of the period also prompted its consumption.

The potato, at its base, is almost certainly a good food (because it is rich in vitamins and minerals) as long as it remains raw. Unfortunately it contains starches that humans are incapable of digesting because, contrary to pigs, they do not produce the appropriate enzymes. That is why we have to cook potatoes before eating them. And while cooking them makes them digestible, it also causes abnormal metabolic effects by breaking down the potato's starches.

All studies done on potatoes for the last twenty years have shown that they have an elevated potential of producing hyperglycemia. The potato is one of the worst "bad carbohydrates" because even the glycemic index of a boiled potato (without the skin) is 70, the equivalent of sugar. But the mode of preparation and of cooking can, as we have seen, cause great variation. It is 90 for mashed potatoes and 95 for French fries or au gratin potatoes.

The index can, on the other hand, be maintained at 65 if the potato is boiled in its skin. It is, moreover, in this form that it was eaten in the past. What is more, at that time it was always served with vegetables, meaning fibers that contributed to lowering the resulting glycemia of the meal.

In our day, potatoes are mostly eaten in their most hyperglycemic forms (fried or baked), and they are generally accompanied by meat, meaning saturated fats. The hyperinsulinism caused by eating them leads to greater weight gain than do the fats eaten during the meal.

Steak and fries, then, is a heresy!

I know what it will cost you to abandon potatoes, but it is the price you will have to pay to reach your objective. When you have attained the result you hoped for, you will not regret it. Know, in addition, that certain deep-fried foods are made with fats that are very rich in saturated fatty acids, which creates a non-negligible cardiovascular risk.

Just the same, it could happen that, as you will see in Phase II, from time to time you might not only not resist a plate of fries, but also deliberately decide to eat potatoes in another form. When you do not have a single ounce left to lose, you can make all kinds of exceptions, but not at just any price. These exceptions will be made during the phase known as exception management.

When you order your meat in a restaurant, right away have the reflex to ask what comes with it because nine out of ten times, you risk finding potatoes on your plate. Ask for green beans, tomatoes, spinach, eggplant, broccoli, cauliflower, or even lentils. And if, unluckily, there are no side dishes without bad carbohydrates, just settle for salad.

At home, when you are deciding what side dishes to serve with meat, you should have the same reflex.

CARROTS
Just like potatoes, the starch in carrots is particularly sensitive to heat. So much so that depending on whether they are raw or cooked, carrots can be considered a "good" or "bad" carbohydrate. When they are raw, carrots have a glycemic index of 35, which is very low. Its consumption in this form can therefore be encouraged. On the other hand, cooking them deconstructs their

starches, which consequently significantly raises their hyperglycemic potential because their glycemic index reaches 85.

Therefore, it is advisable to abstain from eating cooked carrots if you want to succeed at losing weight. Paradoxically, consuming raw carrots, especially grated in a salad, will help you to be successful. Contrary to potatoes, raw carrots are absolutely digestible.

RICE

The most traditional Asian rice (especially long grain) like Basmati has an average glycemic index (50). On the other hand, mass-produced kinds, which have been chosen to be cultivated in Western countries, have high glycemic indexes. The more starch rice contains the higher its glycemic index. This is also the case for precooked rice (index 90).

As with carrots and potatoes, the way rice is cooked can have an effect on its glycemic potential. The longer rice is cooked and the more water it is cooked in, the higher its chances of gelatinizing, a process which causes a rise in glycemic index. This is why rice must always be cooked in the Asian way, which consists of using two parts water for one part rice and leaving the rice to swell after rapidly removing it from the heat.

Just like prolonged cooking, all industrial processing of rice raises its glycemic index. This is true of instant rice (index 85), and rice cakes (index 85). The best way to avoid the breakdown of the starch in rice (which raises its glycemic potential) is to consume brown rice, especially long grain. But this is not always easy to find in restaurants. Indian wild rice, which has nothing to do with real rice because it is a type of oat, can be consumed without any restriction because its glycemic index is very low (index 35).

CORN

Corn is a grain that the indigenous populations of America cultivated for millenniums for food. The original species of corn (Indian), whose varieties are still conserved in agricultural museums, had a low glycemic index (index 35) because they were quite rich in soluble fiber. After the discovery of the New World, Westerners began to cultivate corn for themselves, but even more so to feed livestock. By way of variety selection and hybridism, they were mostly looking to increase output.

Over several years, the glycemic index of corn (modern) practically doubled (index 70). And as we saw earlier for other foods, the starch in corn is so fragile that certain treatments can modify its nutritional structure. That is why making corn into corn flakes or popcorn (two of the most consumed forms in the US) considerably raises the glycemic index from 70 to 85.

Besides the ecological problems created by the depletion of the earth's paretic layers because of the need to abundantly irrigate the modern varieties, the nutritional quality of this industrial corn is quite inferior to that of its ancestors. In Europe we have cultivated corn for centuries, and yet we have only eaten it for a few decades. In the past corn was used almost exclusively to fatten livestock. Fifty years ago, one could not find a can of corn in France because it was a food reserved for animals. It was with the after-war American presence in France that the habit of eating it developed little by little.

PASTA

Everyone knows that pasta is made with white flour. This is why you are most likely waiting for me to advise you to exclude it from your diet. At the risk of surprising you, I will not do this because I have developed the conviction over the years that pasta, at least some of it, is a food that not only will not cause you to gain weight, but on the contrary can help you to lose weight.

But precise explanations are necessary to understand this.

First, you must know that real pasta is inevitably made with durum wheat, while bread is made with tender wheat. The difference is that durum wheat has more protein and fiber (even if the flour is refined), which lowers its glycemic index. Next you must know that certain pasta (especially spaghetti) is extruded. Extrusion is a mechanical process that enables dough to be pressed through openings under very high pressure. The process causes a protective film to develop around the pasta that considerably limits the gelatinization of starches during cooking, but on the condition that the cooking time be as short as possible (*al dente* as the Italians say), meaning five to six minutes maximum.

Let us summarize to assure comprehension. White extruded pasta, because it is made with durum semolina and the process of extrusion, has a low glycemic index (index 50) for an average cooking time (8-12 minutes). If it is cooked longer (12-16 minutes), the glycemic index will go up (index 55). On the other hand, if it is cooked for a shorter period of time (5-6 minutes), the glycemic index will be much lower (index 45).

Finally, chilling pasta lowers its glycemic index even more (a phenomenon of retrogradation). This is why extruded spaghetti made from durum semolina and cooked *al dente* has a glycemic index of 40 if eaten cold, in a salad for example. But clearly if this pasta is whole grain, the glycemic index is the lowest of all (about 5 points less). What has just been said is certainly not applicable to pasta made from soft wheat, and even less for non-extruded pasta. This is generally true for egg noodles, macaroni, lasagna, and ravioli whose glycemic index is high.

This is why you must be extremely vigilant in choosing your pasta. In certain countries like France, pasta manufacturers must use durum semolina. But this is not true elsewhere in northern Europe where a number of pastas offered to the public are made with tender wheat. In addition, whether or not it has been extruded is not easy to verify because the manufacturer is not obligated to put this information on the label. Know that spaghetti is always extruded. On the other hand, tagliatelle is not systematically extruded. The finer it is (and industrially made) however, the greater its chances of being extruded. Be careful just the same with fresh pasta made in certain restaurants (especially tagliatelle and lasagna) which are made from a small manual machine that cuts the strips into a dough previously made by the chef to make a pizza, because it is not extruded.

On the other hand you can consume the famous Chinese vermicelli, made from soy flour (mungo beans) which we know to naturally have a very low glycemic index. Since it is also extruded and only cooked for a few instants, it is the champion of pastas having a very low glycemic index. Therefore, get into the habit of eating spaghetti (the thinnest possible) cooked **al dente** with various sauces (tomato, mushroom, curry) or even in a salad as an appetizer.

LEGUMES

One day, an overweight person told me, "I never eat lentils or beans because my wife says that these starches cause weight gain." On the other hand, he ate a lot of potatoes, which, as you can imagine, did not help matters. He was obviously wrong because certain dried beans can, in effect, contribute to weight loss. This is the case for dried beans, chickpeas, and above all, lentils. Green lentils like split peas even have lower glycemic indexes (22) than green beans.

FRUIT

Fruit is a taboo subject, and if I were to awkwardly dare to say that it is better to eliminate it from your diet, many of you would close this book now, scandalized by such a suggestion. Fruit is a symbol in our culture, a symbol of life, of "richness" and of health. I assure you that we will not eliminate fruit because it is irreplaceable in our diet. But it will be necessary to eat it differently in order to receive all the benefits without experiencing the drawbacks (bloating).

Fruit contains carbohydrates (glucose, saccharide, and especially fructose), but also fibers that lower the glycemic index and therefore diminish the absorption of sugars. Apples and pears are especially rich in pectin (soluble fiber), which helps to limit a rise in glycemia. The energy from fruit is readily usable by muscles and, therefore, is not very susceptible to be stored or accumulated as fats in the body.

But fresh fruit should preferably be eaten on an empty stomach. This particular advice has little to do with the weight loss in which we are interested. It is instead to assure better digestive comfort because the consumption of fruit at the end of a meal, as is often the habit, can cause digestive problems. Elderly people are especially sensitive, children much less so. For adults it all depends on the sensitivity of the individual. But let us try to understand why.

The digestion of fruit begins in the mouth with the chewing and ends in the small intestine. Fruit, then, has nothing to do in the stomach but go through it. When fresh fruit is eaten after foods containing proteins, such as meat or cheese, it is blocked for a certain amount of time in the stomach by the digestion of the proteins even though it would prefer to pass quickly to the intestines. Fruit is imprisoned in the stomach and, under the effects of heat and humidity, may ferment, sometimes even causing a small amount of alcohol to be produced. The whole digestive process could then suffer (bloating).

Fruit, then, must be eaten by itself! This is a rule that we should probably teach at school. School-age children's bodies can react more easily. But adults, and especially the elderly, should definitely not eat fruit at the end of a meal. But when, then, should you eat it?

Whenever you have an empty stomach – in the morning for example, before breakfast. But you should wait about fifteen minutes before beginning to eat something else, in order to allow it to pass easily through the stomach. You could also eat fruit late at night before going to bed, that is, at least three hours after the end of dinner. A piece of fruit could also be eaten in the middle of the afternoon. But you should also be sure to leave a sufficient amount of time following lunch (about three hours) and before dinner.

As all rules have exceptions, some kinds of fruit, because they have a very low concentration of sugar, do not ferment easily. Included in this category are strawberries, raspberries, black currants, red currants, and blackberries, which can be eaten with no problem at the end of a meal.

Cooked fruits can also be eaten at the end of meals because they lose the ability to ferment in the stomach. You must not forget, however, that cooking them causes them to lose most of their vitamin C. Lemon does not ferment either, so you can drink its juice (unsweetened) at any time or use it to flavor food (on fish or in salad dressings).

I will end this section by making one additional suggestion. Whenever possible, also eat the skin of fruit, after having properly washed it. The skin is rich in fiber, and it is often within that the greatest concentration of vitamins is found. Eating fruit (preferably organically grown) it its skin lowers the glycemic index even more. You will lose weight even more effectively if you respect this rule.

Among the important "foods", we still must discuss beverages, the first of them being alcohol.

ALCOHOL

Alcohol causes weight gain. This is what you think because it is what you have been told. Perhaps you have even been made to feel guilty by people who tell you that your extra pounds are caused by the alcohol you drink regularly. We are going to objectively sum up the issue.

It is true that alcohol can contribute to weight gain if it is drunk in excessive quantity. But if you remain reasonable, it can be neutral. In the weight loss stage, you should limit your consumption to a small glass of wine (4 1/2 ounces) at the end of the meal. But in order to obtain the best results, it would be better to completely eliminate even this small amount in order to avoid further temptation. Once weight loss is obtained, you will see that it is absolutely possible to drink two or three glasses of wine a day without compromising your weight.

Alcohol provides energy that is almost completely used by the body. During this time, the body will tend to not burn stored fats. It therefore puts weight loss on hold. But this happens mostly when alcohol is ingested on an empty stomach. When the stomach is already full, especially of proteic lipids (meat, fish, and cheese), alcohol metabolizes much more slowly and contributes little to the production of stored fats.

On the other hand, you must consciously eliminate before-dinner drinks. If you feel you absolutely must join your guests, have something non-alcoholic like tomato juice or sparkling water with a slice of lemon. The only noble cocktail, in my opinion, is a glass of good champagne or sparkling wine. But please, do not allow the addition of black currant liqueur or any other strange syrup (usually added to mask the mediocrity of a poor quality wine or champagne). If you cannot do otherwise, accept a glass of good champagne at cocktail time, but above all, **do not drink on an empty stomach.**

Begin first by eating a few appetizers. But be careful to choose appetizers without bad carbohydrates. You will quickly learn to recognize them. In this category, avoid chips, crackers, and finger sandwiches. Acceptable appetizers are olives, cheese, cold cuts (dry salami for example) or fish (smoked for example). Two or three small pieces of cheese and a slice of dry salami are enough to close the pylorus (a sphincter found between the stomach and the small intestine) slowing down the passage of alcohol into the blood.

Just the same, in Phase I you should try to completely eliminate cocktails because it is a rigorous Phase in which the basic rules of the Method must be applied painstakingly in order to bring about weight loss.

After dinner drinks (digestifs)

As for digestifs, cross them out. Cognac, Armagnac and other brandies may be delicious (if you can stand them), but not at all good for reaching your ideal weight. Maybe you only drink digestifs because you really think they help you to digest. Believe me, once you have adopted the dietary principals contained in this book, you will no longer have any problem with digestion, even after a copious meal.

Beer

Beer is also a beverage that should be consumed with moderation. It is not necessary to travel to Germany to know that the side effects of beer are bloating, weight gain (especially if drunk between meals), bad breath, indigestion despite the presence of diastase, small enzymes whose role is precisely that of activating digestion. One must be prudent with beer because it contains both alcohol and even more importantly, a carbohydrate (maltose) whose glycemic index is very high (index 110). The combination of alcohol and sugar promotes the hypoglycemia that causes fatigue and therefore, under-performance (see Chapter 6 on hypoglycemia). That is why, if you are a heavy beer drinker, you would do better to decide to drink much less, especially between meals. During meals, you should drink no more than 20 cl (8 ounces) maximum, remembering that your weight loss will be greater if, in Phase I, you decide to give it up completely.

Wine

We have already discussed wine, but it is worth it to come back to it because there are interesting, even positive, things to say about it. Since the beginning of the 1980s, numerous scientific studies have shown that wine (especially red) has incontestable medicinal virtues, but also certain preventative virtues. It was notably shown that a moderate, regular consumption of wine[12] could be an efficient factor in lowering the risk of cardiovascular diseases. These studies, leading to the concept of the "French Paradox," showed, in effect, that if the French had three times less risk of having a heart attack than Americans, it was precisely because they drank eleven times more wine.

More recently (1995), it was proven that the most beneficial property of wine was its content in the powerful antioxidants,

---

[12] *Michel Montignac's* The Miracle of Wine *("Boire du vin pour rester en bonne santé") is to be published in the US soon.*

polyphenols. Moreover, it was even shown that some of these polyphenols, taken in through moderate wine consumption, could prevent certain cancers and even Alzheimer's disease.

But what interests us the most is that wine consumption can be the cause of your being overweight. We have already said that excessive quantities of wine (alcohol) could contribute to weight gain. Two to three glasses a day should, on the other hand, have no real effect. A small glass of wine (4 ounces) at the end of a meal could even, according to some experts, have positive effects on insulin secretion. If you have enough will power to limit yourself to small amounts, your weight loss will be more significant. The rest of you should abstain from drinking wine during the entire first Phase of weight loss.

In Phase II, as we will see later, wine will be able to be consumed daily without jeopardizing weight maintenance. Drinking wine should just the same be carefully managed along with other sources of carbohydrates.

When you begin Phase I, where you must stick firmly to the Method's principals, it may be difficult to participate in a family meal or an outing with friends without drinking a drop of wine. If you announce right away that you are not drinking, it could be uncomfortable for the others.

My advice is the following: allow your glass to be filled and pick it up as often as if you were normally drinking. Wet your lips with it instead of drinking at as you normally would. In short, pretend, which I grant you is not easy.

I personally practiced this method for several weeks and believe me, no one ever noticed that I was not "participating". In the same way, no one ever noticed that I did not eat a single crumb of bread. To fool people, I always take my piece of bread, but it stays on the table. I never really "touch" it.

To end, I emphasize that the amount of alcohol in vinegar is completely negligible. It can therefore be used to flavor raw vegetables and salads, unless you prefer lemon.

COFFEE

Real coffee, well-ground Italian espresso, is not, as some believe it to be, dangerous. Because of the pressure it goes through, the amount of caffeine is not necessarily high, even if it has a strong flavor. In fact, filtered coffee made the American way is the most problematic because even though it is thought to be weak (because it is clear like tea), it still contains a great deal of caffeine.

If you wish to succeed at your weight loss program, you must not take any chances. Therefore it is important to know that, even though caffeine is not a bad carbohydrate, it is not any less capable of causing a slight rise in insulin secretion, especially for those who are highly hyperinsulinic. That is why I would advise you to "slow down" on coffee and even to eliminate it during this first stage.

If you are a heavy drinker of very strong coffee, it is most likely because you feel you need a stimulant to keep you awake. If you regularly have sudden drowsy spells, especially around 11:00 a.m. or in the afternoon when you are digesting your lunch, it is because you are experiencing the effects of hypoglycemia (see Chapter 6). So drink decaffeinated coffee, or at least pure Arabica coffee, which contains much less caffeine.

Excessive coffee consumption , like that of sugar, cigarettes, or alcohol, comes from a kind of dependence that has developed over the years. It is therefore worthwhile to break this cycle once and for all. If your motivation to obtain substantial weight loss is strong enough, you will do your best to stick to the necessary resolutions. Once you have obtained the results that you were looking for, and your pancreas has gone back to its normal working state, you will be able to, from time to time, (in Phase II) to finish off a good meal, allow yourself to enjoy a good espresso.

SOFT DRINKS

These drinks are generally made from synthetic fruit extracts or plants, and all have the same major disadvantage: they contain a lot of sugar (index 70). They are, therefore, objectionable and, because of this, to be totally excluded, not only because they contain a lot of sugar, but because their artificial carbonation causes aerophagia.

Even if made from natural extracts, you must beware of soda, which can be toxic. In effect, significant amounts of hazardous substances, like terpenes, can be found in natural citrus extracts. The worst soft drinks are colas. They should either be strictly prohibited or carry special warnings such as those found on cigarette packs: "This product is hazardous to your health." Unfortunately, cola consumption has spread to every country in the world.

I leave it to Dr. Emile-Gaston Peeters to comment on the subject. "Right now, the cola sold on the European market contains, for 19 cl (average amount of a small bottle) around 21 mg of caffeine and 102 mg of phosphoric acid. Caffeine has stimulating properties. Phosphoric acid is intensely acidic and its high phosphorous concentration can upset the body's calcium/phosphorous ratio, which can lead to a serious calcium deficiency in the bones. Finally, you must make certain that the phosphoric acid used does not contain high amounts of toxic heavy metals. The conclusion is simple. Cola must be, in its present composition, **formally discouraged** for children and adolescents. It does not benefit anyone."

This declaration obviously needs no commentary. Whether for your children or for yourself, the firm recommendation is the same: no soft drinks, no sodas, and especially no cola.

MILK

Whole milk is a complex food because it contains proteins, carbohydrates (lactose) and fat. As we will see later, milk fat is bad (saturated). That is why it is better to drink skim milk. Powdered skim milk is, in my opinion, quite preferable because if you add a larger quantity of powder than what is normally recommended, you can obtain an unctuous liquid rich in proteins, which can serve as a supplementary aid in weight loss. But among all the dairy products, it is best to opt for sugar-free yogurt (plain or low-fat), taking advantage of the numerous healthy qualities of its active cultures.

FRUIT JUICES

What was said earlier about fruit is also true for fresh fruit juice, meaning the juice obtained immediately after having pressed the fruit. Its glycemic index is higher than the fruit from which it comes for the simple reason that it lacks pulp, meaning fiber. That is why, instead of drinking fruit juice that can elevate glycemia (except lemon), it would be better to eat fruit instead during the weight loss Phase. As for commercial fruit juices, even if they are "pure fruit" without added sugar, they are lower in vitamins and fiber than fresh fruit juices. In addition, they contain too much acid. They should only be consumed on exceptional occasions.

THE APPLICATION OF PHASE I: WEIGHT LOSS

The first Phase of our Method is not difficult to put into practice. But in order to truly succeed you must have a complete grasp of the basic concepts of the system. And based on my experience, it is at this level that some may encounter failure.

This is not to question your intellectual ability to integrate a new concept. However, I am asking you to give up predisposed notions that are so engrained in our subconscious that they reveal veritable cultural conditioning. The relatively simple ideas and the "elementary" scientific principals introduced here have unfortunately not yet gone further than the walls of certain enlightened researchers who are ahead of their time[13]. So you should not count on society to help you in your undertaking. In addition to respecting the major metabolic principals you discovered in the preceding chapters, it would also be good, in order to be as efficient as possible, to apply good-sense rules.

One is that it is imperative that you <u>never skip a meal</u> (especially lunch) because that could disturb the body, which will be tempted at the next meal to make abnormal reserves. You must eat three meals a day, with perhaps a snack. Eat a copious breakfast, a normal lunch, and a light dinner. Because the same food, especially if it is fatty, is more "fattening" in the evening than in the morning. Putting Phase I into practice is dependant upon a fundamental principle of the Method and two rules of application:

1) The fundamental principle: to make dietary choices that lead to a resultant glycemia that is as low as possible at the end of a meal so as to keep insulin production at a minimum.

---

[13] The fundamental principles of the Montignac Method were confirmed by the result of epidemological studies by Professor Walter C. Willett of The Harvard School of Public Health's Department of Nutrition in Boston.

2) The rules of application: two types of meals are possible. Either the meal will be mostly proteic-lipidic (meat and fish for example) and will only contain carbohydrates with a <u>very low</u> glycemic index (less than or equal to 35) like green lentils, chickpeas, green vegetables, etc. Or the meal will mostly be glucidic-proteic. It will thus contain <u>no</u> saturated fat and <u>very few</u> poly- or monounsaturated fats. The carbohydrates will be chose from among those whose glycemic indexes are lower than 50.

BREAKFAST

Breakfast #1
It will contain few fats and lots of carbohydrates having a low glycemic index (GI). You can eat one or more pieces of fruit as soon as you wake up, then begin your breakfast around fifteen minutes later. You can use this time to get dressed or watch the morning news.

1st option: consists of mostly fiber-rich bread (whole wheat, but preferably <u>real</u> integral whole grain bread).

No standard exists for this; each baker, in fact, is free to use his or her own recipe. That is why "whole wheat" bread often has nothing whole about it except its name because it is generally the result of a mixture of white flour with a "certain amount" of material retained during refinement. But whole wheat bread can also simply be made with a lesser-refined flour. Bran bread comes from a mix of white flour and a specific amount of bran.

Here again, there is no standard indicating **what percentage must be in the bread in order to have the right to name it.** Added bran, in addition, is often made from wheat obtained through an intensive, modern, agro-industrial process; that is, there is a significant chance that it contains residue from pesticides. Therefore, I advise you to choose only <u>real</u> whole grain bread, (fresh or toasted), which, I must say is not always easy to find. More and more natural food stores[14] are selling it.

Real whole grain bread conserves the "integrality" of the components of the wheat grain, which makes it a "good" carbohydrate with a low glycemic index. It is richer in fiber, proteins, minerals, trace elements, and B vitamins. You can also by German bread (*schwarzbrot* or pumpernickel) that can sometimes be found in large stores, but study the label well because they often contain sugar and saturated fats (palm oil).

Optionally or simply to vary your pleasure, you can also eat whole wheat crackers <u>rich in fiber</u> or containing oats (grains rich in soluble fiber). In any case, it is best to exclude all forms of classic bread, which, besides being made with white flour, generally contains bad fats and sugar.

But what will you put on your whole grain bread? It is naturally preferable in Phase I to not eat butter or margarine, even though we will eventually be able to do so in Phase II. Above all, do not use honey because its glycemic index (GI) is high (index 90), or classic jam, which contains 65% sugar. I suggest two options.
- You can use sugarless fruit marmalade, meaning fruit pulp jellied with pectin and guaranteed sugar free. Even though the taste is close (even without added sugar) it is nothing like classic jam. The glycemic index (GI) of this product is low, which makes it an excellent accompaniment to whole grain bread.
- Or you can use fat free cottage cheese or plain yogurt, which you can eat alone or flavored with sugarless marmalade, or even salt or pepper. The difference in fat content between a low-fat yogurt and a plain yogurt is 1.2 g per 100 g, which is very little.

---

[14] *To have a complete list of stores selling products chosen by Michel Montignac, call* 1-877-333-7422 *or write to Erica House, P.O. Box 1109, Frederick, MD 21702. E-mail: info@MontignacUSA.com*

2nd option:

The Phase I breakfast can also be composed of unrefined cereals chosen with the greatest of care because they should not contain sugar, honey, caramel, corn, puffed rice, etc. Granola having these characteristics may also be eaten. Unrefined cereals (oats, granola) may be consumed with skim milk (hot or cold) or even mixed with plain yogurt. You can even add a little bit of sugar-free marmalade if necessary.

At all costs you should avoid cereal made with refined flour, the most common ones containing puffed rice (index 85) or those made with refined corn flour, like the all-too famous corn flakes (or rice flakes) whose glycemic index is 85. All Bran can, on the other hand, be integrated in small amounts because it is very rich in fiber; unfortunately, it contains sugar. Naturally, it is possible to have a combination of whole grain bread and unrefined cereal. To end, let us specify that it is absolutely acceptable to have fruit for breakfast, adding a skim milk product and yogurt in order to obtain a sufficient amount of protein

Breakfast #2
This breakfast will be mainly *proteic-lipidic* and, therefore, salty. It can be composed of ham, bacon, cheese, or eggs (scrambled, soft-boiled, or fried). It is an American-type breakfast. However, in Phase I, it should contain no carbohydrates, to avoid raising insulin levels in the blood and causing the body to store fat.

So no toast, even if it is whole grain. This is the ideal formula when at a hotel where fiber-rich bread and unrefined cereals are practically non-existent, or else on the weekend when you have a little more time to make it.

This breakfast is not advisable, on the other hand, for those who wish to exercise in the morning because the absence of carbohydrates at breakfast does not prepare the body well enough to do intense physical exercise. Just the same, it is important to only sometimes have this particular breakfast because it is high in saturated fat. It is completely unadvisable for those who have high cholesterol or general cardiovascular problems.

Since this breakfast is low in carbohydrates, except for the lactose from the milk or perhaps some yogurt, it would be wise, in light of a balanced diet, to think about what else you will be doing throughout the day. That means that the other meals in the day will have to be rich in "good" carbohydrates and low in bad fats (saturated).

Breakfast beverages

Your breakfast beverages, no matter which food option you choose, should be chosen from the following options:
-decaffeinated coffee (or coffee containing little caffeine like Arabica)
-weak tea (otherwise it can contain too much caffeine);
-chicory (alone or with coffee);
-skim milk (the powdered form can provide a thicker, more concentrated mixture).

During Phase I, you must avoid chocolate flavored drinks (children could drink a sugar-free, non-fat mix). All of these beverages should be consumed without sugar. You could use an artificial sweetener (like aspartame) or a little fructose, but try to wean yourself from the taste of sugar.

LUNCH

Lunch, whether eaten at home or out, will most often be made up of proteins, lipids, and carbohydrates with a very low glycemic index (GI). Proteins essentially come from meat, fish, eggs, and dairy products.

Lipids will either be those generally associated with proteins or those that are added during food preparation (like olive oil). Your choice of fats will be particularly important in preventing cardiovascular risk.

The carbohydrates that will be eaten during the meal will be chosen exclusively from among those whose glycemic index (GI) is less than or equal to 35, which you found listed on p. 41 and which will be touched on in the following pages.

THE TYPICAL LUNCH MENU WILL BE THE FOLLOWING:
- raw veggies or soup (hot or cold)
- fish, meat, or poultry
- side dishes (carbohydrates with a GI less than or equal to 35)
- salad
- cheese or yogurt,
- beverage: water, optionally 4 1/2 ounces of red wine or 8 ounces of beer at the end of the meal.

Starters

All salads are allowed, as long as none of its ingredients contain bad carbohydrates. Verify before ordering that there will be no **potatoes, corn, cooked carrots, or beets** in your salad. Raw vegetables can be seasoned with olive or sunflower oil, and vinegar or lemon.

If you are in a restaurant, you may have bacon bits on your salad. Yet you must be sure to specify when ordering your salad with bacon bits: **without croutons** because most restaurants have the unfortunate habit of adding them.

Be vigilant. Do not begin to tolerate "small errors" that are, in fact, enormous, considering your objective. Let your server know how particular you are. If you asked for "no croutons" or "no corn" do not be complacent by accepting "just this once" because he or she is busy.

If you want the waiter/waitress to take you seriously, you must be convincing by insisting on the fact that "it would be absolutely unacceptable for you to find the slightest trace of what you do not want in what you are served." Personally, I have found that the best way to have your wishes respected is to say that you are allergic. This works every time. As long as you find green beans, leeks, artichokes, cabbage, cauliflower, tomatoes, endives, asparagus, mushrooms, radishes, cheese, meats, or even lentils, chickpeas, or dried beans, you can eat as much as you would like. Exclude from this list of hors d'oeuvres red beets (their index is 65) and, as we have already said, corn.

As for eggs, there is no restriction, even with mayonnaise.[15] Yes. A little mayonnaise, just like a little bit of light sour cream is completely acceptable because we are not concerned with their caloric content. This does not mean you can go crazy with them. If you like them, eat normal amounts. But if you have high cholesterol, it is best to be careful and avoid them altogether (see Chapter 8). For an appetizer, you can also have tuna, sardines in oil, crab, prawns, or smoked or marinated salmon.

The main course

The main course will be composed essentially of meat, poultry, or fish, accompanied by a vegetable. There is no restriction to make in this category, except in the preparation, even though it is best to choose fish, being that its fats are much more effective in preventing cardiovascular risk. We also know that fish fats are not nearly as easily stored as the others are. Some studies even show that they aid in weight loss.

---

[15] If the mayonnaise is from a jar, verify its ingredients. It is highly possible that it will contain sugar, glucose or flour.

Meat and fish should never be fried with batter because the coating is a very bad carbohydrate, which in addition soaks up bad fats. Similarly, fish should never be rolled in flour (or breaded) before cooking. Get in the habit of always asking for grilled fish. Also avoid cooking and frying fats. They are not always easily digestible, and they increase cardiovascular risk.

Be careful of sauces. If you are accustomed to "nouvelle cuisine", the sauces are normally quite light, as long as they do not contain flour. Most of the time, they are made from the cooking juices and a bouillon or light cream. In traditional cooking, sauces are usually thickened with white flour (high GI), which is dangerous according to our principles.

If you are eating good grilled meat, you can eventually use a béarnaise sauce, as long as you do not have cholesterol problems, because it contains butter and egg yolks. If you use mustard, avoid the sweet kind because it contains sugar.

As far as side dishes, you will most often choose fiber-rich vegetables. From tomatoes to zucchini, to green beans, egg plant, cauliflower, broccoli, or lentils, you will have the burden of choosing. Refer to the complete list on page 114.

As I advised you before, if nothing else is available when you are out to eat, and only bad carbohydrates are offered, then simply eat lettuce. Green and red loose leaf, frisée (fine, curly endive), escarole, dandelion greens, and romaine are all acceptable. You can also eat as much of this as you would like, as an appetizer, the main course, and before or with the cheese.

Cheese

Eating cheese at the end of a meal is a very French tradition. Even if you are in a country that has different eating habits than the French, which is the case in the US, nothing can stop you from eating them if you enjoy it, and if you are still hungry after the main course. But you will have to get into the habit of eating cheese without bread because, even if <u>real</u> (integral) whole grain bread is available, its glycemic index will be more than 40. It is not worth it to take useless risks in Phase I.

The best thing to do is to enjoy your cheese with a green salad. As another technique you can use a firm cheese like Swiss or Cantal as a base for a softer cheese. All cheese is allowed in Phase I. But you can also end this type of meal with yogurt or cottage cheese. Remember that you should never eat too much cottage cheese (some people have the tendency to end all of their meals with it). Some authors have said that milk proteins contain growing factors or even weight gain factors necessary to fatten up small veal, but also active in humans. That explains why eating too much of a dairy product can hinder weight loss.

In addition, some people, especially the elderly, cannot digest dairy products well because they are lactose intolerant. They lack an enzyme called lactase that is necessary to the digestion of lactose. This intolerance, which is not an allergy, can cause fermentation and uncomfortable bloating.

Dessert

The big problem with classic desserts is that they almost always contain three major ingredients: white flour, sugar, and butter. Some "Montignac" desserts can be made from cooked fruit (apples, pears, apricots, peaches), eggs and fructose, a "natural" sugar whose glycemic index is low. But they can also be made from bitter chocolate containing more than 70% cacao. I have included extensive recipes for these desserts without bad carbohydrates in my different cookbooks (also see Appendix). But their consumption is more reserved for Phase II.

In Phase I, you can, once in a while, Sundays for example, have dessert with your meal as long as you are sure that the carbohydrates with which they are made have a glycemic index less than or equal to 35. Some desserts can be made with artificial sweeteners, as long as they do not need to be cooked for a long time, in pudding or custard for example. I prefer fructose. It works better in baking because it has the same consistency as sugar and tolerates heat better.

Beverages

We have already said that it is best to avoid all alcoholic beverages, in Phase I unless you are able to limit yourself to a small glass of red wine (4 ounces) or beer (8 ounces) at the end of a meal (never on an empty stomach). So drink water, weak tea, or herbal teas if you like them. In any case, you should drink very little during your meals because you will drown your gastric juices, slowing down digestion. Whatever you do, only begin to drink during the second half of the meal. Avoid drinking as soon as you sit down. This is a bad habit that too many of us have gotten into. Rather, drink between meals (at least 1.5 quarts). But think about it. We too often forget to do it.

If you are obligated (professionally, for example) to eat large meals during Phase I, let me remind you that you must avoid the alcoholic cocktail. Have tomato juice or mineral water. If you absolutely must accept an alcoholic beverage (a punch, for example, was made for everyone and is automatically given to you) take it, but do not drink it. Wet your lips with it from time to time in order to "participate", but do not consume it. At the opportune moment, you can "forget it" somewhere without anyone noticing. In some circumstances it will be more difficult for you to get rid of it. In that case, challenge your imagination. Put it in the path of heavy drinkers who always manage "distractedly" to take over other people's drinks, especially when the glasses are full. If this type of person is not around, which would be surprising because they are normally everywhere, you still have flower pots, the champagne bucket, the window in the summer, or the lavatory sink.

IF YOU MUST GO TO A RECEPTION WHILE YOU ARE IN PHASE I, HERE IS SOME ADVICE:

As you know, you can accept a glass of champagne if it is handed to you. Keep it for a while, then discretely put it down somewhere. The food served at a reception is always a problem. But there is no problem without a solution. Naturally, it is out of the question for you to eat finger sandwiches, no matter how small they are, because they are made in part from "bad carbohydrates." On the other hand, what is on the sandwiches is often quite acceptable: slices of salmon, salami, egg, asparagus, tomato, etc. If you are astute enough to separate the middle from its bread base, bravo!

Nothing is impossible when you are motivated. And there is always food at a reception that is in total agreement with our rules of eating. **Look for the cheese.** There is often cheese in some form or another. Eat it sliced or in little cubes. Otherwise, look for sausage or cocktail wieners.

If you do not think you will be able to resist such a display of food, if you think that you will have to succumb because you are hungry and you cannot control yourself, here is a solution: snack on something filling before you go to the reception.

In the middle of the nineteenth century, my great-great grandfather, who had six children, was once a year invited to have lunch with his family at the home of the head of the company for which he worked. My great-great grandmother, so was reported to me, took great care on that day to have all six children eat a hearty soup before going that day. Being fairly full, the charming children showed a much less excessive enthusiasm for eating exceptional dishes that they were never served at home. And my great-great grandparents acquired a reputation for having extremely well raised children.

If you are afraid of not being able to resist the abundance of food on a buffet, eat a hard-boiled egg or a piece of cheese before the reception. You can even get into the habit of taking those small, individually wrapped cheeses with you. These little "just-in-casers" can also fulfill the little hunger pang you may have at the end of the morning or in the afternoon. Fruit, like an apple, that is rich in fiber would be even better.

Except for children, for whom snacks are necessary, if your meals are well planned and sufficiently rich in protein and fiber, you should not be hungry between meals. In any case, never confuse these "just-in-casers" with a snack or nibbling.

If you are invited to eat at a friend's home, your choices will obviously be more difficult, as your chances to "maneuver" the situation will be significantly decreased. Let us look at the situation from all its angles. These friends may be people you know well. They may even be family members. So take advantage of the freedom you have with them to discretely "tell them how it is." Ask beforehand what they will be serving, and do not be afraid to make suggestions.

If you are not at all close to your hosts, you will have to do what you can at the last minute and improvise. If this invitation is "exceptional", what is served at the meal will correspond. It would therefore be surprising to see rice, corn, or potatoes served.

If there is **foie gras**, eat it without a second thought because it is completely acceptable, with the good fats it contains. But please **do not eat the toast on which it is served which is surely made from white flour.** No one will force you to eat it. Not even propriety.

If you are served a magnificent cheese soufflé, eat it just like everyone else, even though it contains flour. But do not let yourself go. Do not make the situation worse by having second or third helpings.

If the appetizer is a a paté in a crust shell, eat the inside, which is generally proteic-lipidic, and discretely leave the rest in a corner of your plate. If you are not in familiar company, no one will be impolite enough to say to you, "Look, you're leaving the best part." Even if she asks herself the question silently, your hostess will not ask you why "you didn't like her crust."

As far as the main dish is concerned, I do not think you will have any problem with the sides, which are generally varied. At a dinner, it is rare that only one vegetable is served. That is why, besides the potatoes that you are not obligated to take, there will surely be green beans, broccoli, mushrooms, or another vegetable that is "acceptable" for you. But if everything is served directly on your plate, the choice will be more difficult. In any case, no one will force you to eat what is on your plate.

If after that you are still hungry, catch up on the salad and especially the cheese if there is some. If you compliment the hostess on her cheese, she will appreciate it and forgive you more easily for having left the crust of her paté. Great cheese trays have an extensive display of different types. Guests normally do not take much because, after all the bread (white) they have eaten, they no longer have room for cheese. So honor the tray.

Dessert is obviously a critical moment because it is always difficult to say, "no thank you, I do not want any." So insist on just a **very small piece** and do as those who are not hungry any more, leave a good-sized part on your plate.

Finally, wait as long as possible to begin to drink. Drink red wine if possible, especially with the cheese. But limit yourself to the very minimum.

If the situation was even worse than what you thought it would be, if you absolutely were not able to escape the attack of the bad carbohydrates, even though you are right in the middle of Phase I, you simply must be even more vigilant in the future when it comes to putting your new eating principles into practice.

Because you must know that in Phase I, you are still very fragile. As long as your pancreas has not experienced a long period of rest, it will still be tempted to respond to any indulging with excessive insulin production. That is why if, all at once, you introduce a large quantity of bad carbohydrates into your body after having completely deprived yourself for some time, you take the chance of suddenly going back to where you were when you started. That can be completely discouraging. Tell yourself just the same, as you would in other circumstances, that a battle lost does not ruin your chances of winning the war.

DINNER

Dinner will be:
- either identical to lunch but lighter, meaning limiting your consumption of fat and replacing it with vegetables,
- or proteic-lipidic like breakfast, meaning mainly composed of "good" carbohydrates, avoiding saturated fat intake (meat, butter, dairy products, etc.) and keeping your intake of poly- and monounsaturated fats to a minimum (a vinaigrette on your salad at the most). Because fats eaten at dinner are the most easily stored. Nocturnal hormonal activity and an inactive nervous system facilitate the makeup of stored fats. Fats eaten at dinner (particularly saturated fats) have a greater chance of being stored than the same fats had they been consumed during the first part of the day.

Dinner #1:

Just like for lunch, it can be composed of a starter, a salad for example, raw vegetables, or a soup containing only "good carbohydrates". The main dish will be made up of proteins and lipids (meat, fish, eggs) accompanied by a vegetable found on the list of carbohydrates with a very low GI. The biggest difference between lunch and dinner is that dinner is most often eaten at home, which can be both good and bad. It is inconvenient because at home the choices are always more limited. Also, most of the time, you eat with your family at home, and the menu is the same for everyone. But if you are able to convince your family and share the recommendation with them, you should have no problem.

The ideal would be to begin the evening meal by a thick vegetable soup. In this soup you can use leeks, celery, cabbage, etc. It should be made exclusively of vegetables that are very low on the GI scale. Be careful. The cook may be tempted to use potatoes. This cannot happen. Potatoes can make the soup consistent, but celery can also play this role. There is another way to bring together vegetable soup. That is to add egg yolk or several mushrooms puréed in the blender. Moreover, it has been shown that soups containing large pieces are more effective in weight loss than those that are too liquid. Escape from instant soup, because of what they are made of, they have a high GI.

In the evening, it is better to avoid eating meat, unless it is poultry. Instead, eat fish because, as we have already seen, the fat from fish is much less readily storable. Some studies even say that it encourages weight loss. Avoid meat in the evening, especially if you ate beef, veal, lamb, or pork at noon. This would be too large an intake of saturated fats for one day. These fats are both more liable to be stored and, in excess, likely to raise your cholesterol level.

As for a dairy product, cheese is always welcome, and it is good to alternate it with yogurt, which we know to have important nutritional value. We know, in effect, that it helps to balance intestinal flora. It was even recently discovered that it helps to lower cholesterol, reinforce resistance to infection, and fight constipation. But be careful. Only eat good yogurt, without artificial flavors or sweetened fruit. To be sure, buy plain or organic yogurt.

Since you most often eat dinner at home, at least take the opportunity to eat simple, permitted foods that you enjoy. Like stew (with the fat skimmed off), mackerel, or sardines. Eat things that you never find in restaurants like boiled artichokes. They are delicious, rich in minerals, and contain a lot of fiber, which improves intestinal transit and lowers glycemia. Above all, do not forget to eat vegetables, tomatoes, spinach, endives, eggplant, cauliflower, leeks, zucchini, broccoli, and mushrooms, that you can prepare in different ways, steamed for example, and that you can combine to make up an entire dish (ratatouille).

Dinner #2

This second dinner is by far the one that will provide the best results when it comes to weight loss. Like your breakfast, it will mostly be composed of carbohydrates having a very low GI and protein, and it will contain very little fat (absolutely no saturated fats and a minimum of poly- and monounsaturated fats).

For this meal, you can choose from among the following:
- vegetable soup (without potatoes or carrots)
- brown rice with a tomato sauce
- pasta, more specifically spaghetti cooked al dente (whole wheat is best), which you can accompany with a tomato and basil or herb sauce
- lentils seasoned with onions
- red or white beans
- whole wheat semolina with vegetables
- artichokes with an olive oil vinaigrette

For dessert there is always cottage cheese or yogurt, plain (its fat content is negligible) or low fat, whose flavor can be enhanced by a sugar-free fruit marmalade. You can also eat cooked fruit (apples, pears, apricots, peaches, etc.) because it does not at all have the same effects as raw fruit (it does not ferment). This is why it can be eaten at the end of a meal.

Have this Dinner #2 two, three, or four times a week, even every day if you wish. It will permit you to rebalance your diet by opting for good carbohydrates, especially legumes (lentils, beans, chickpeas, etc.), which contain vegetable proteins.

To maintain a varied spread of main courses for one week, it is best to eat:
- Three times per week: meat
- Three times per week: poultry
- Once to twice per week: eggs
- Three to four times per week: fish
- Three to four times per week: "good" carbohydrates (whole grain foods, legumes), besides those you use as side dishes for the other main meals listed above.

Starches with low glycemic indexes (lentils, beans, peas, chickpeas, pasta, and brown rice) not only **can** be included with dinner, they **must** constitute a large portion of the meal.

Too many people hesitate to follow this recommendation because they still think, "Starches cause weight gain." In fact, no. As we said before, there are "good" and "bad" starches. You just have to choose.

Remember, adopting the Montignac Method first means setting aside any preconceived ideas. Therefore, if carbohydrates are part of the list of low-glycemic index foods, especially very low-glycemic index foods, you must eat them; not only as side dishes, but also as the main part of the meal.

FAST FOOD

At this stage, I am convinced that you no longer even think of the ham sandwich your favorite deli makes, or worse yet, the infamous fast-food hamburger on a horrible little white bun. Fast food is nevertheless a practical response to the new organization of our society. It is just unfortunate that most of the food stuffs that are favored the most in fast food restaurants have a high, or very high, glycemic index.

For several decades, because of the official recommendations of nutritionists Americans have been obsessed with fat, which they have tried to take out of all their food. The food industry, therefore, has attempted to take out the fat while preserving the taste, or even to replace the fats with substitutes. If that did not do much for the fight against obesity, since fats were not the main cause, it at least proved that the food industry was still capable of ingenuity.

As soon as those in charge have understood that the enemy is not so much fat as it is bad carbohydrates, there is no doubt they will be capable of concocting fast food whose carbohydrates will be chosen exclusively from the low and very low glycemic index column of carbohydrates. This does not mean that it is not important to pay attention to the nature of fats as well (see Chapter 8).

But while you wait for this to happen, you can invent an acceptable fast food for yourself. We can, for example, make a "Montignac sandwich." First of all, the bread absolutely must be real (integral) whole grain bread. You can even toast it because doing so reduces its glycemic index.

Between the two slices of integral bread, you can put whatever low-glycemic index carbohydrate you want, avoiding all fats except fish or even olive oil. Very lean meats (chicken or turkey breast) are also acceptable.

But instead of the sandwich made on whole grain bread exclusively garnished with the ingredients listed above, it is always possible to bring one's lunch in a cooler. The lunch could consist of a dish made up of the previously listed foods, especially chicken breast, Swiss cheese, tuna, raw vegetables, and even lentils, etc. If you are not able to prepare your lunch beforehand, you can always improvise by buying everything you need at the last minute in a small convenience store.

For example, you can buy:

-   Ham (cooked or smoked): I recommend this because it always comes in thin slices that can you can eat without a fork or knife.
-   Dry sausage (as low in fat as possible): but you will need a knife. A letter-opener will do the job.
-   Hard-boiled eggs: you can find these easily in delicatessens.
-   Tomatoes: if you are sure to have a good supply of tissues or paper towels nearby, tomatoes are ideal.
-   Cheese: any cheese will do, but we must, in this case, stay practical. I would exclude cheeses that are not easy to handle because they "run" for example, or because they have a strong odor that your close neighbors would not appreciate, especially if

Examples of possible components of a real multi-grain bread sandwich		
Artichokes	Dijon mustard	Chicken breast
Cucumber	Fat-free cheese	Cooked ham
Green pepper	Fat-free cottage cheese	Herring
Lettuce	Plain or fat-free yogurt	Smoked salmon
Mushrooms		Tuna in water
Onion		Turkey breast
Puréed green lentils		
Puréed chickpeas		
Raw carrots		
Tomato		

you are on public transportation. Therefore, make your selection from among Swiss, cheddar, and other firm cheeses.

Naturally, all of this will be eaten without bread, even whole-grain bread.

If your stomach is completely empty, you could, as I already told you, make up your meal of fresh fruits (especially apples and pears) or dried fruits (apricots and figs). Eat as many as you need to fill you up. The bad thing about fruit is that it is digested very quickly. That is why it is ideal to eat it with something more consistent containing protein – almonds, hazelnuts, or walnuts for example, or even yogurt.

SNACKS

If you correctly follow the principals of the Method and if your lunch is filling enough, you should not feel the need to eat before dinner. However if at the end of the afternoon, you feel a stubborn pang of hunger, it is best to eat something. Above all, never go for the prohibited bad carbohydrates like crackers, chips or popcorn, or even worse, pseudo-chocolate bars and other snacks. Instead, eat two apples or else dried fruit, preferably apricots or figs, or even wrapped cheese. You can even have yogurt with a little sugar-free "marmalade."

If you exercise at the end of the day, fifteen minutes before doing so you can eat fruit (fresh or dried). The muscles you use will immediately use up the energy from good carbohydrates.

OTHER RECOMMENDATIONS

Now we are approaching the end of the explanations necessary to putting Phase I into practice. If, before adopting these principals, you normally ate sugar, were a great admirer of sweets, and ate large quantities of white bread and lots of potatoes, you could lose eight to ten pounds in the first month.

Above all, do not stop there by going back to your old bad eating habits because the same causes produce the same effects, and you will most likely rapidly regain what you have lost. You must avoid constant weight fluctuation at all costs. After this first period, weight loss will continue, provided you scrupulously adhere to my recommendations. Your weight loss should thus follow a continuous rhythm, even though the amount is completely individual.

For some people, it will definitely happen more quickly than for others. Experience shows that rapid results often are obtained more easily in men than in women, except maybe for those who are hyperactive or undergoing particular medical treatments (some medicines can cause weight gain).

In effect, excess weight in men is almost exclusively due to hyperinsulinism. Women are subject to a larger hormonal influence, which may also affect their weight. But this does not mean that the results will be less noticeable. Some women have had more trouble obtaining results than others have.

Four possible causes have been identified:
- anxiety, which stimulates insulin secretion;
- hormonal perturbations during adolescence or menopause;
- thyroid problems, which are rather rare;
- some women's bodies establish a special form of resistance, at least at first, due to previous food deprivations from following excessive and repeated low-calorie, abusive diets. Some of these diets can even cause a multiplication of fat cells. (To learn more about resistance to weight loss, see Appendix III).

If you have had cholesterol problems in the past, there is no reason to worry now. Experience has shown that eating carbohydrates having a low glycemic index and choosing good fats, as I recommend doing in this book, has led to normalization in a large majority of cases. It is especially important to avoid saturated fats, which may raise cholesterol, instead choosing fats that lower bad cholesterol and raise good cholesterol.

Finally, these ideas are positively acknowledged by all the world-specialists, and the scientific publications in this field are numerous (see Chapter 8 on hypercholesterolemia). Although it is highly improbable, your doctor may not agree with this new dietary approach because it does not correspond with what he or she learned in medical school. Remember, in this field like in others, new ideas may be slow to evolve, despite irrefutable scientific proof that contradicts traditional thinking. In any case, know that <u>there is no danger in following the principals of my Method.</u>

What risk could there be in consuming foods that are natural, unrefined, rich in fiber and micro-nutrients (vitamins and minerals) that our ancestors ate for millions of years before us? How could we be stupid enough to support the idea that the consumption of high-glycemic index foods (sugar, refined flour, potatoes, modern high-yield hybrid species, and industrially treated products) is better for our health? Such an assumption corresponds to the same strange thinking (or even mental debility) that assumes that it is healthier to live in the polluted atmosphere of a big city than in fresh, country air.

If some people criticize you, not understanding your new dietary choices, let them go ahead. Let them be astounded by the results that you are sure to obtain. Not only will you lose weight, but you will also improve your blood chemistry.

If you regularly respect the rules of Phase I, it will be impossible for you to not see results. If, if fact, that is the case, or if weight loss takes an abnormally long time, it is because something is not being done correctly (see Appendix III). Therefore, for a while you should keep a list, an exhaustive list, of everything you eat from morning to evening. By keeping this dietary journal, you will be able to find that which is not in keeping with the principals we have just covered. You could, for example, be eating too much yogurt, or even regularly eating soup that you have been told only contains "authorized" vegetables such as tomatoes, sorrel, leeks, etc., when, in fact, that is not the case.

Always be suspicious, and verify what the ingredients actually are. Most famous soups come in a can or package. If you read the label, you will notice with amazement that in addition to the authorized vegetables, the soup also contains bad carbohydrates in the form of thickening agents such as modified starches. So be careful. Even if our dietary principals are not difficult to put into practice, they demand, at least in the first Phase, a certain effort and, let's face it, some sacrifice. Do not risk making foolish compromises.

But watch out. If you are currently following (or recently followed) a low-calorie diet, do not move too quickly to the application of this Method. Your rational body still remembers its recent frustrations. An abrupt reintroduction of larger amounts of food could possibly cause your body to store fat. It is then possible that you could gain three to five pounds before beginning to lose weight. In order to avoid useless weight gain, begin by applying the Method, increasing quantities progressively until you come to a normal level of satiety.

If you are at the end of a low-calorie diet, or if your diet was poorly balanced, you may notice (only in the beginning of the Method) that your weight will not change even though your body is getting thinner. You feel that you are losing weight, and yet your scale is not showing it. The explanation is simple. It is merely because you are in the process of regaining your muscular mass. You are, in fact, losing fat but gaining muscle. Muscle takes up less space than fat, but it weighs more.

Finally, if you had a diet very low in fiber before, do not incorporate large quantities of it all at once. Add it progressively so your intestines can become used to it. The colon's flora will thus progressively adapt, providing for good digestion of this higher amount of fiber (unrefined foods, legumes, fruit, vegetables, raw veggies, etc.). At first, you may experience bloating, slight abdominal pain, even very soft, frequent stools.

DURATION OF PHASE I

The legitimate question you will probably ask at the end of this chapter is: how long must I stick with Phase I. I will respond with a phrase often used by a late great French comedian, "For a while." It depends on many different things.

Phase I should last as long as it takes to lose your excess weight, keeping in mind that weight loss usually progresses on an individual basis. You could also say that the end of Phase I corresponds to the attainment of your ideal weight. Chapter 12 explains this calculation.

But instead of talking about ideal weight, we should instead talk about fitness weight, or balanced weight, a very individual idea that corresponds to the attainment of a threshold beyond that around which the body has decided to stabilize and stop weight loss.

If you have twenty to thirty pounds to lose, Phase I could last several weeks to several months. If you only have ten to twelve pounds to lose, you might be tempted to stop as soon as you have attained your goal. But let me remind you that the goal of Phase I, besides getting rid of excess pounds, is above all to <u>re-balance the functioning of your pancreas in order to allow it to raise its threshold of tolerance for glucose</u>. This takes at least two to three months.

Consequentially, if you prematurely cut back on Phase I, even if you have lost enough weight, you may not yet have given your pancreas enough time to become healthy. Hypothetically, if you have no weight to lose and are following the Method solely to gain more physical and intellectual vitality, the problem obviously remains the same. You should prolong your Phase I for as long as possible to re-harmonize all your metabolic and digestive faculties for good.

Realistically, you should not even have to think about the length of Phase I because the switch to Phase II will not happen overnight, but rather quite progressively. You will notice that Phase I is not at all constraining because you do not have to limit yourself quantitatively. You will also notice that you will feel so good that you may even have trouble leaving this Phase.

LET US SUMMARIZE THE MAIN PRINCIPLES OF PHASE I

- Eat until you are full (to satiety), without quantitative restriction or counting calories. But do not consistently overeat.
- Eat three meals a day at specific times, and never skip a meal.
- Avoid eating between meals. An eventual snack is acceptable in the late afternoon if it permits you to eat a lighter dinner.
- Your meals must be structured and varied.
- The dietary balance among the three principle nutrients (carbohydrates, lipids and proteins) must be attained each day, but each and every meal should necessarily contain both carbohydrates and proteins.
- Breakfast will be centered on good carbohydrates containing little or no fat.
- Lunch will contain proteins, fats and carbohydrates, but the carbohydrates must have a very low glycemic index (less than or equal to 35).
- Dinner will be:
    - Either identical to lunch, but lighter and with few fats,
    - Or it will essentially be made up of carbohydrates. In this last case, an effort should be made to use very low GI carbohydrates

(less than or equal to 35) if the meal contains saturated fat. If the fat contained in the meal is reduced to a minimum and this minimum is composed of mono- and/or polyunsaturated fat, you may use low GI carbohydrates (less than 50).

- Limit your consumption of saturated fats (meat, fatty cold cuts, butter, and whole dairy products), and instead opt for fish fats and olive or sunflower oil.

- Avoid all sweetened beverages.

- Do not drink more than one glass of wine (4 1/2 ounces) or beer (8 ounces) with any one meal.

- Avoid coffee that is too strong; get in the habit of drinking decaffeinated.

- Take your time while eating. Chew well and avoid tension during your meals.

CONCLUSION OF PHASE I

In this first section, we discovered two new categories of carbohydrates: "good" ones that we can eat without fear of gaining weight and "bad" ones that we must watch for and systematically avoid. The difference between them is in the intestinal absorption of glucose, which depends on several things:
- Fiber content
- Protein content
- Cooking time, which causes the gelatinization of starch
- Industrial processing.

This is why the more flour is refined, the higher its glycemic index and the greater the body's insulin response will be, sometimes to excessive levels. The excess insulin then causes the body to store the fats contained in the meal.

In the same way, the longer a potato is cooked at high temperatures (fried or baked), the more its glycemic index goes up. The same is true among other starches, including those that normally have a low glycemic index. It is true for lentils (index 22 to 30) which, when cooked to the point where they form a thick, gelatinous cream (as is done frequently in India), can end up having a high glycemic index of 60 to 70.

As you have already seen, the idea of a glycemic index is basic to the Montignac Method. You understand that if we gain weight (especially if we become obese) it is because we are hyperinsulinic. And that if we are hyperinsulinic it is because our glycemia at the end of meals is much too high. And if we periodically experience hyperglycemia, it is because our diet is too hyperglycemic, which is due to the fact that the carbohydrates we consume have glycemic indexes that are much too high.

Remember, that for close to half a century, nutritionists and other dieticians have been on the wrong path. They have been stressing the "quantitative" nature of foods, recommending that overweight people lower their caloric intake, even though today we are discovering that it is the "qualitative" nature of foods that makes the difference.

You learned in the earlier chapters that there are "good" and "bad" carbohydrates, some of which cause weight loss and others weight gain, by producing different metabolic reactions. In the same way there are "good" and "bad" fats, some indirectly raising cholesterol, others precisely lowering it (see Chapter 8).

Before going to the tables summarizing what we have just learned, I would like you to think about the wonderful hope the Montignac Method has to offer all those desperately fighting extra pounds. With what could easily be described as the "dietetics of failure" because of its low-calorie nature, one always had to consume fewer and spend more and more calories, and with practically no results.

With the principles of the Montignac Method we come to realize that there is a veritable reversibility in the metabolic pathology that represents obesity. By eating normally, but judiciously choosing our foods, we can finally lose our extra pounds for good, attain better general health and especially enjoy life more.[16]

---

[16] To understand the results obtained by weight loss based on the Montignac Method, read Appendix V on page 223 where you will find scientific studies on the topic.

PROTEIC LIPID SALTED BREAKFAST

	Recommended	Acceptable	Prohibited
Fruit*		Apples Strawberries Raspberries Lemon Apricots	Preserves Canned fruit cocktail Bananas Chestnuts
Eggs		Eggs over-easy Soft-boiled eggs Omelet Scrambled eggs	
Fish	Smoked salmon Smoked trout Herring Shrimp		
Meat		Bacon Sausage Smoked ham Cooked ham	Hotdogs
Cheese		Fermented cheeses Fresh cheeses Yogurt	
Bread **Pastries** **Cereal** **Sweets**		Only with fish: - Whole wheat toast - Fiber-rich cracker Avoid bread when eating saturated fats: - Meats - Eggs - Cheese	All bread All cereals All pastries All cakes Sugar Honey Maple syrup
Beverages	Skim milk Decaffeinated coffee Weak tea Hot chocolate	2% milk	

*To imperatively be consumed 20 minutes to 1/2 hour before the rest of breakfast.

"GOOD" CARBOHYDRATE-RICH BREAKFAST

	Recommended	Acceptable	Restricted
Fresh fruit*	Apples, pears, oranges, lemon, grapefruit, kiwi, peaches, grapes, nectarines, cherries, plums, strawberries, raspberries	Pineapple Papaya Mango	Bananas Chestnuts
Bread Pastries Cakes and Sweets	Multi-grain bread	Whole wheat bread Pumpernickel bread Rye bread Whole wheat toast Whole wheat bagels	White bread Croissants Pancakes Brioche Muffins Biscuits Waffles Sugar Honey Maple syrup
Cereal and Grains Yeast	Sugar-free whole grain cereals Oat bran Wheat germ Beer yeast	Sugar-free granola Oatmeal Wheat bran	Sweet cereals Cornflakes Puffed rice Popcorn
Preserves	Sugar-free marmalade Sugar-free applesauce	Preserves made with fructose Sugar-free peanut butter	Preserves Jellies Sweetened peanut butter
Dairy and soy products	Fat-free or plain yogurt Fat-free cottage cheese Plain soy yogurt	Full-fat yogurt Low-fat cottage cheese	Sweetened full fat yogurt Fruit yogurt Sweetened soy yogurt
Beverages	Powdered skim milk Decaffeinated coffee Weak tea Low-fat hot chocolate Soy milk	Fresh fruit juice Vegetable juice 2% milk	Sweetened fruit juice Soda Cola Alcohol Whole milk Chocolate milk mix

*To be consumed imperatively 15 minutes to 1/2 hour before the rest of breakfast.

EXAMPLES OF GOOD CARBOHYDRATE BREAKFASTS

Fresh orange juice Peach	Fresh carrot juice Orange	Grapefruit/ orange juice Kiwi
Multi-grain bread Sugar-free marmalade Fat-free yogurt	Oatmeal Preserves made with fructose Dried fruit Fat-free yogurt	Sugar-free granola Oat bran Wheat germ Fat-free cottage cheese
Decaffeinated coffee Powdered skim milk	Tea Powdered skim milk	Weak coffee Powdered skim milk

Fresh apple juice Raspberries	Orange juice/ lemonade Pear	Apricot juice Prunes
Multi-grain bread Butter/ olive oil Fat-free yogurt Wheat germ	Whole wheat toast Sugar-free applesauce Fat-free yogurt Beer yeast	Fiber-rich crackers* Sugar-free peanut butter Soy yogurt
Coffee Powdered skim milk	Coffee Powdered skim milk	Weak tea Powdered skim milk

*Without sugar or palm oil

EXAMPLES OF PROTEIC-LIPIDIC BREAKFASTS

Fresh orange juice Apple	Fresh carrot juice Raspberries	Fresh apple juice Strawberries
Smoked salmon Multi-grain toast Tomatoes Cucumbers	Soft-boiled eggs Lean smoked ham Lettuce Tomato	Scrambled eggs Lean cooked ham Fermented cheese Mushrooms Tomatoes
Coffee Soy milk	Tea Milk	Decaffeinated coffee Powdered skim milk

BALANCED PHASE I MEALS (LUNCH OR DINNER)
WITH VERY LOW GLYCEMIC-INDEX CARBOHYDRATES

APPETIZERS			
VEGGIES	FISH	MEAT*	OTHER
R E C O M		M E N D E D	
Asparagus	Smoked salmon	Dry sausage	Mozarella
Tomatoes	Marinated salmon	Smoked ham	Baked chèvre
Cucumbers	Sardines	Cooked ham	Sweetbreads
Artichokes	Mackerel	Salad with bacon bits	Frogs' legs
Green peppers	Herring	Salad with giblets	Escargot
Celery	Anchovies	Liver paté	Omelet
Mushrooms	Tuna	Foie gras	Hard-boiled eggs
Green beans	Cod liver		Fish soup
Leeks	Shrimp		
Heart of palm	Scallops		
Cabbage	Prawns		
Cauliflower	Lobster		
Gherkins	Caviar		
Avocado	Shellfish		
Soy germ	Crab		
Quinoa	Calamari		
Lettuce	Cuttlefish		
Endives	Oysters		
Frisée	Crayfish		
Dandelion leaves			
Watercress			
Broccoli			
Radishes			
Raw carrots			
Lentils			
Dried beans			
Chickpeas			
P R O H I		B I T E D	
Carrots (cooked)		White sausage	Puff pastries
Beets		Terrines made with	Quiche
Corn		flour	Pancakes
Rice			Soufflés
Tabbouleh			Toast
Potatoes			Croutons
Pasta			Pizza
			Dumplings/Donuts
			Cheese fondue

*In order to prevent cardiovascular risk, meats should be chosen according to their saturated-fat content (see Chapter 8).

BALANCED PHASE I MEALS (LUNCH OR DINNER)
WITH VERY LOW GLYCEMIC-INDEX CARBOHYDRATES

MAIN COURSE			
FISH	MEAT	POULTRY	OTHER MEATS*
R E C O M		M E N D E D	
Salmon Mackerel Tuna Sardines Herring Bass Cod Red mullet Trout In general all salt- and freshwater fish	Beef Veal Pork Lamb Mutton	Chicken Hen Guinea fowl Turkey Goose Duck Quail Pheasant Pigeon	Hare Venison Wild boar Andouilles Black pudding Ham Beef heart Kidneys Pigs' feet
R E S T R I C T E D		T O B E A V O I D E D	
Fried fish	Fatty cuts	Skin	Too-frequent consumption

*To prevent cardiovascular risk, you should choose meats according to their saturated-fat content (see Chapter 8).

PHASE I MEALS ACCOMPANIMENTS (LUNCH-DINNER) WITH VERY LOW GLYCEMIC-INDEX CARBOHYDRATES

SIDE DISHES	
RECOMMENDED	**RESTRICTED**
Lentils	Couscous
Chickpeas	Chestnuts
Split peas	Cooked carrots
Dried beans (white)	Rice
Green beans	Turnips
Broccoli	Cooked broad beans
Eggplant	Squash
Zucchini	Rutabaga
Spinach	Gnocchi
Mushrooms	Corn
Celery	Millet
Sorrel	Pasta
Endives	Noodles (macaroni)
Leeks	Ravioli
Tomatoes	Lasagna
Onions	
Green peppers	
Ratatouille	
Cauliflower	
Cabbage	
Sauerkraut	
Green lettuce	
Artichokes	

MISCELLANEOUS INGREDIENTS

Condiments, ingredients, seasonings, and diverse spices				
TO BE CONSUMED:				RESTRICTED:
PREFERABLY in normal quantities			In reasonable quantities (not to be abused)	
Gherkins Pickles Baby onions Homemade vinaigrette Green olives Black olives Celery salt	Oils: - olive - sunflower - peanut - walnut - hazlenut - grapeseed Lemon Parmesan Gruyère	Parsley Tarragon Garlic Onion Shallots Tyme Bay leaves Cinnamon Basil Chives Anise	Mustard Salt Pepper Mayonnaise Bearnaise Hollandaise Cream sauces	Potato starch Corn starch Ketchup Industrial may- onnaise Floury sauces Sugar Caramel Palm oil Paraffin oil Maltodextrine Modified starches

EXAMPLES OF "BALANCED" PHASE I DINNERS WITH
VERY LOW GI CARBOHYDRATES

Homemade lentil soup	Fish soup
Over easy eggs	Cooked ham
Ratatouille	Green salad
1 yogurt	Cheese
Split pea soup	Artichokes in vinaigrette
Stuffed tomatoes	Smoked salmon
(see recipe in Appendix)	
Green salad	Green salad
1 yogurt	
Onion soup	Leek soup
Tuna flan	Cold chicken breast, mayonnaise
Green salad	Green salad
Cottage cheese	Cheese
Endive salad	
Cucumbers in light sour cream	Asparagus
Turkey breast	Poached filet of white fish
Tomato sauce with basil	Spinach
Yogurt	Cheese

Beverage: water, weak tea, herbal tea, 4.5 oz. wine or 8 oz. beer

PHASE I CARBOHYDRATE DOMINATED DINNERS
(FAT FREE*)

Homemade vegetable soup Brown or wild rice with tomato sauce 1 plain yogurt	Homemade vegetable soup Whole wheat spaghetti with tomato sauce Fat-free cottage cheese	Grated carrots Chickpeas with tomatoes Sugar-free applesauce
Lentils with onions (fat-free sour cream sauce) Green salad with lemon juice 1 low-fat yogurt	Baked tomatoes with parsley Dried beans (fat-free sour cream sauce) 1 plain yogurt	Mushroom soup Brown rice with tamarin Low-fat yogurt
Whole wheat couscous with vegetables (GI<50) (without meat or oil) Fat-free sour cream-based sauce+harissa+cumin +several pinches of bouillon	Cucumber salad Eggplant stuffed with mushroom purée and fat-free sour cream 1 low-fat yogurt	Lentil soup Quinoa with tomato sauce Baked apple

Beverage: water, weak tea, herbal tea, 4.5 oz. wine, or 8 oz. beer
*Except a bit of olive oil.

PHASE I CARBOHYDRATE DOMINATED DINNERS:
(RICH IN FIBER)

	Appetizers	Main courses	Desserts
Choice of Carbohydrates	Vegetable soup Cream of mushroom soup Lentil soup Tomato soup Etc.	Lentils Dried beans Peas Chickpeas Brown rice Whole wheat semolina *Al dente* spaghetti	Fat-free cottage cheese Fat-free yogurt Applesauce Stewed fruit Sugar-free marmalade
Recommendations	Without fats, potatoes, or cooked carrots	Without fats (except olive oil and fish), served with tomato sauce mushroom sauce, or vegetables	Sugar- and fat-free

EXAMPLES OF PHASE I MENUS
"BALANCED" LUNCHES WITH VERY LOW GIs

Tomato salad Veal chop Green lentils Cheese	Cucumber salad Filet of cod (tomato sauce) Peas Yogurt
Radishes Turkey breast Puréed chickpeas Cheese	Walnut endive salad Grilled ground beef patty Broccoli Yogurt
Quinoa taboulleh Filet of salmon Au gratin zucchini Cheese	Hearts of palm Pork cutlets Puréed celery root Yogurt
Leeks in vinaigrette Grilled kidneys Salsify Cheese	Grated carrots Leg of lamb Dried white beans Yogurt
Sardines in oil Spicy sausages Cabbage Cheese	Asparagus in vinaigrette Grilled black pudding Puréed cauliflower Yogurt
Frisée Grilled game hen Broccoli Cheese	Meat bouillon with fat skimmed off Stew Leeks and cabbage Yogurt
Smoked salmon Duck Mushrooms with parsley Mixed greens with cheese	Tuna in olive oil Steak tartare Mixed greens Yogurt
Red cabbage Ray with capers Puréed green beans Cheese	Grated carrots Grilled salmon Spinach Yogurt
Tomatoes and mozarella Grilled chicken Green beans Cheese	Artichoke hearts in vinaigrette Rib steak Eggplant Yogurt

Beverage: water, weak tea, herbal tea, 4.5 oz. wine, or 8 oz. beer

Chapter 5

THE METHOD, PHASE II WEIGHT MAINTENANCE

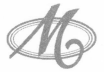

Learning Phase II will take us back to the basic principles of the Method. In order to understand this maintenance Phase in the best way possible, we must place it in the general context of the metabolic effects that are linked to the glycemic potential of your meals. The previous chapters explained that the resulting glycemia of a meal (postprandial glycemia) is responsible for setting off the process of the storage of the fats eaten during that meal.

Let us remember that the resultant glycemia is the average rise in glycemia at the end of a complex meal because of the interaction between the different foods of which it was composed. A sweet, for example, will cause glycemia to rise, while fiber-rich vegetables, on the other hand, will help to lower it if you ate high glycemic index foods earlier (potatoes, for example).

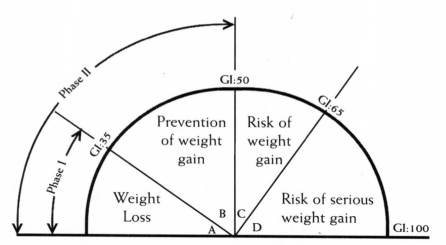

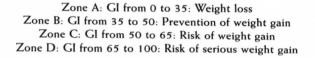

Amplitude of the rise of weight gain and chances of weight loss based on the resultant glycemia of a meal according to the Montignac Method

Zone A: GI from 0 to 35: Weight loss
Zone B: GI from 35 to 50: Prevention of weight gain
Zone C: GI from 50 to 65: Risk of weight gain
Zone D: GI from 65 to 100: Risk of serious weight gain

As this chart shows, if the resulting glycemia of a meal is between 65 and 100, there is a strong possibility of weight gain (obesity). This is what explains the high level of obesity in countries like the United States, where the majority of foods consumed have a high glycemic index (sugar=70, French fries=95, hyper-refined flour=85, and corn flakes and popcorn=85). If the resulting glycemic index of a meal is between 50 and 65, hyperglycemia will be lower, but still significant enough to constitute potential weight gain.

This situation is probably that of the French, Italian, and Spanish. Even though such populations also consume high-glycemic index carbohydrates (potatoes, white flour, and sugar), they couple them with foods having a low glycemic index (green vegetables, lentils, beans, chickpeas, fruit, spaghetti, etc.). The resulting glycemia of their meals is thus just slightly above average, creating less of a potential for obesity. When obesity does occur it is less extreme, but still a concern.

To lose weight, the resulting glycemia of a meal must not be above 35. That is the only way the secretion of insulin will be low enough to inhibit lipogenesis (the storage of excess fat) and stimulate lypolysis (the breakdown of stored fats). This is what we were doing during Phase I by limiting our choices of carbohydrates to those whose glycemic index is very low. This is how, without concerning ourselves with caloric intake, we were able to begin losing weight.

Phase II consists of weight maintenance, meaning cementing the substantial weight loss you obtained in Phase I by only consuming carbohydrates with a very low glycemic index. Of course you could stay in Phase I for your entire life. The advice you have been given provides a perfectly balanced, nutritionally rich diet. The people who do this have discovered such well-being in Phase I that they never want to stop.

Even though Phase I must remain a permanent nutritional reference, it excludes certain foods that are generally part of our normal diet. Of course it leads to the attainment of a sort of "metabolic ideal," but its relative integration can be too limiting to allow you to continue a normal social life, especially a gourmet social life. When you follow low-calorie diets, you rapidly begin to maintain a conflicting relationship with food, which you begin to consider the enemy little by little. Anorexia is one of the most severe consequences of this.

The Montignac Method, however, reconciles us to food. But its true goal is to go even further. The Method will turn you into a true gourmet (if you were not one already). Eating should be considered one of the supreme values of existence. This is why cuisine is a veritable art, just like music or painting, an art that fits everyone, that symbolizes the quality of life to which we aspire. Cultivating this art not only means making yourself aware of the vital importance of food but, above all, of the sensory pleasures we receive in discovering different foods and various preparations. It would be a pity to forever deprive yourself of foods that, despite having critical metabolic effects, have excellent gastronomic qualities.

When I was little, my parents took me two or three times a year to the circus and four or five times a year to the movies. Each time, like for all children (good children) of the time, they bought me a chocolate ice cream. Ice cream has no real, positive nutritional characteristics if we analyze its composition (sugar and saturated fat). Consuming a dozen per year like we did at the time had no consequences. Although it had no nutritional value, it had emotional value. Today, most Western families' freezers are full of ice cream. We eat it practically every day. In a country like the United States, it is eaten much more often than that.

In the same way, 100% of fast food or other average restaurants systematically serve fries with their main course. In most cases, even if you say that you would like something else instead (like a salad), they bring them to you anyway. That is how difficult it is for the personnel to go against this practice, which reveals the systematization of the typical restaurant industry.

In a 1994 article in a gastronomic review, I "nailed" a Parisian restaurant that, despite its star in the Michelin Guide, offered au gratin potatoes as the only side dish in ten out of twelve of their menu's main course options.

Eating an ice cream, a plate of potatoes, or even a piece of pie from an excellent bakery from time to time never hurt anyone. But if you eat those things every day, or worse yet more than once every day, then you should not be surprised that you will experience some undesirable side effects. As Hippocrates so rightly said, "it is the amount (and the frequency) that makes the poison."

You learned in previous chapters that if the greatest number of overweight people and diabetics are found among the American population, it is unfortunately because their consumption of high-glycemic index carbohydrates is permanent. The problem in America, which is progressively becoming a problem throughout the world, is that the consumption of unhealthy foods (having a high glycemic index) which should have remained occasional in order to be acceptable, has since become regular and systematic.

The Montignac Method proposes nothing **but a re-balancing and re-centering of eating habits** based on these criteria.

Contrary to what some people mistakenly believe, Phase II is not about periodically, for several days or even for several weeks, going back to the old, unhealthy eating habits you may have had before beginning the Method. Then, after having regained several pounds, rigorously going back to Phase I, your body could accept this game of yo-yo three or four times, but it would develop resistance to the point where Phase I would no longer have the same efficacy.

This is often true of those who, having taken in the first three-quarters of the book, only applied some of the principles without trying to understand them, and especially without resituating them in a global nutritional vision. Others did even less, considering Phase I was just a regular "diet" whose only merit, in their eyes, was that it was the most efficient and least tedious. Once they had lost weight, they stopped applying the principles overnight, beginning to eat hyperglycemic foods again, just as they did before.

The host of a famous French television program once told me, before walking onto the set of the show to which he had invited me, "I tried your diet, Montignac, and I have to say that it is easy and very effective. The only bad thing is that as soon as you stop, you rapidly gain the weight back." I responded that based on principle, the same causes produce the same effects, and it seemed logical to me that he would gain back the weight by again eating white bread, sugar, and potatoes at every meal.

"Why didn't you do Phase II?" I asked him.

He looked at me, astonished, and told me he did not know what I was talking about. In fact, he had never read my book. He had only applied the several select principles outlined in a brash summary he had found on a page he had gotten from one of his journalist friends.

This is why you must first understand the basic principles of the Method in order to enjoy long term success with Phase II. Phase II can be followed in two different ways — with or without exceptions. In both cases, the goal is the same: **to end up with a glycemic index that does not go above the average (50) by the end of the meal.**

PHASE II WITHOUT EXCEPTIONS

This way consists of <u>broadening Phase I</u>. Phase II is in some ways a continuation of the first one.

Let us remember that in Phase I, for proteic-lipidic meals (that is, those containing meat, eggs, whole dairy products, and diverse fats) the carbohydrates eaten with them must imperatively be chosen from among those with a very low glycemic index (less than or equal to 35). Phase II without exceptions will allow you to broaden your range of possibilities by consuming now and then carbohydrates with a glycemic index less than or equal to 50. For example, you will be able to eat Basmati rice (index 50) or *al dente* spaghetti (index 45) from time to time with fish. You will also be able to drink orange juice (index 40), eat kidney beans (index 40) or even sweet potatoes (index 50).

During meals, you will be able to drink more than one glass of wine (two or three are possible) or even an entire bottle of beer (12 ounces) without any danger of changing your weight. Your average glycemia, even if it slightly increases, will still be low enough to stop any excessive insulin secretion capable of causing eventual weight gain.

Obviously, all additional recommendations I made before should still be applied, especially those that consist of opting for good fats (olive and fish oils) and limiting your consumption of saturated fats, particularly in the evening.

PHASE II WITH EXCEPTIONS

This way is more complicated because it is subtler. It will consist of permitting the <u>exceptional</u> consumption of high-glycemic index carbohydrates, but <u>only under certain conditions</u>. This means that each time you eat a food having a high glycemic index, you must absolutely compensate for it by introducing an opposing food. In other words, if you eat a food that raises glycemia, like potatoes, you will be strictly obliged to eat something else that will help to lower the resulting glycemia (see figure I on next page).

In the second half of the nineteenth century in Europe, the consumption of potatoes was much more widespread, especially among poor populations and peasants. Most of them ate potatoes every day yet still were not fat. The explanation is simple.

First, the potatoes they ate were almost always cooked unpeeled in water or ashes, which *a priori* causes only a small rise in glycemia (index 65, compared to fries and au gratin potatoes whose index is 95). In those times, potatoes were almost always the main ingredient of a hearty, thick soup containing a number of vegetables and thus, fiber. In France, potatoes were most often

FIGURE I

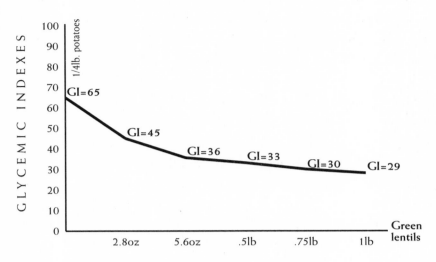

Evolution of the theoretical resultant glycemia of a meal composed of 1/4lb of boiled, unpeeled potatoes (index 65) compared to different amounts of green lentils (index 22).

consumed with cabbage. In Spain, they were eaten with lentils.

Each time the people of that time ate potatoes (high GI), they also ate large quantities of foods with a low glycemic index at the same time. The resulting glycemic index was, therefore, average. In the same way, it may surprise you that even though the glycemic index of rice is above average (depending on the type, it varies between 50 and 70), the Chinese have never been obese. The explanation is the same as that of our potato-eating ancestors.

In the Chinese diet, rice (a carbohydrate with a rather high GI) is always eaten with vegetables whose glycemic index is very low because they are rich in fiber. The resulting glycemic index of their meal is, therefore, well below 50.

In Phase II, this is exactly what we must concern ourselves with: no matter what we eat, we must arrange it so the resulting glycemia of our meal will be as low as possible. Obviously, this calculation will never be precise because not only would you have to measure every carbohydrate eaten, but also have access to a computer to make all the necessary calculations. Experience shows that all this is not really necessary because we can succeed simply by applying a few of the basic rules. But to understand the principles, you first must learn several fundamental notions.

Since the beginning of this book, you have been learning that, contrary to what we thought for a long time, <u>not all carbohydrates are equal</u>. In effect, some have high glycemic potential, like potatoes, while others, on the other hand, have low glycemic potential, like lentils. But what you also must know is that their pure carbohydrate content is different.

In a baguette, pure carbohydrates account for 55% of the product. They make up 33% of fried potatoes, 49% of potato chips, 14% of boiled, unpeeled potatoes, 17% of lentils, only 6% of cooked carrots, and a mere 5% of lettuce and broccoli. In order to compare comparable things, the calculation of the glycemic indexes was done "at equal pure carbohydrate quantities".

Therefore, we can compare the index obtained from consuming 3.5 oz. of sugar with that of 10.5 oz. of fries, 7 oz. of chips, 1.25 lb. of lentils, 1.5 lb. of boiled potatoes, or 4.5 lb. of lettuce. All of these portions are comparable according to their glycemic index because they all have something in common: they contain 3.5 oz. of pure carbohydrates.

The goal of Phase II, as we already noted, is management of exceptions, but two parameters complicate the process slightly:
- the glycemic potential of the carbohydrate, measured by its glycemic index, and
- the food's pure carbohydrate concentration.

1. The glycemic index of the carbohydrate:

This is a notion you now know well. To tell the difference between high-glycemic index carbohydrates and low-glycemic index carbohydrates, simply refer to the table (page 41). In Phase I the choices were simple because each time you wanted to eat a carbohydrate, you chose from those whose index was very low (35). In Phase II we are still going to keep our eyes on the table of glycemic indexes because, even if we feel we can allow some exceptions, our goal must be to limit the incidence of this as much as possible.

For example it is understandable for you to want to eat potatoes sometimes. The table of glycemic indexes will help you to limit the consequences of your exceptions. By opting for potatoes boiled in their skins (GI 65), you will certainly be making an exception, but it will remain controllable. The more your exceptions are modest in their glycemic consequences, the easier it will be to compensate for them.

Having made an exception, you still have to decide how you will make up for it. Common sense will tell you that if you choose to compensate with a carbohydrate having a glycemic index of 40 (like kidney beans) you will have trouble making the resulting glycemia add up to 50 or less. That same common sense will lead you to choose compensation carbohydrates from among those whose glycemic index is lowest instead. Logically, you might think that the lower the glycemic index, the greater the compensatory effect. You might also think that any green vegetable with a GI lower than 15 would be an ideal choice. In fact, you will be right as long as the pure carbohydrate concentration is the same. As we saw earlier, this concentration differs from carbohydrate to carbohydrate.

2. The pure carbohydrate concentration

The glycemic index of a carbohydrate is important, but it must be associated with its pure carbohydrate concentration. You will notice in the table on p. 138 that carbohydrates have different pure-carbohydrate concentrations. In traditional dietetics, the carrot was considered to be on the same level as all other carbohydrates: potatoes or lentils, for example. So, besides the differences we noted in terms of glycemic potential, it is also important to note the differences in pure-carbohydrate content from one product to another.

First, there can be differences within the same family of carbohydrates, as with potatoes. We have already noted that their glycemic indexes vary according to the way they are cooked. We also know that the pure-carbohydrate concentration also varies according to the same parameters.

Cross-checking the glycemic index table with that of the pure-carbohydrate concentration, then, can reveal good and bad surprises.

Among the good surprises, we can note that cooked carrots, whose glycemic index is critical, only has a weak pure carbohydrate concentration (6g per 3.5 oz.), which is just a little higher than that of lettuce. We can then establish that choosing to make an exception by eating cooked carrots will have very little glycemic consequence, especially if you eat only a small amount. For the glycemic consequence to equal that of a baked potato, you would have to eat four to five times more carrots; six times more to equal French fries. In other words, you would have to eat about 1.3 pounds of cooked carrots to induce the same critical result in glycemia as do 3.5 oz. of fries.

The conclusion you may draw is that in Phase II you no longer have to be as obsessed with cooked carrots as you were in Phase I. If you come across a couple of slices of these colorful little carbohydrates, eat them without feeling guilty or even wondering how to compensate for them. The same process can be applied to all carbohydrates with a high glycemic index whose concentration in pure carbohydrates is weak or very weak, especially turnip (3%), pumpkin (7%), watermelon (7%), cantaloupe (6%), and beets (7%). If you do not eat them often or in great quantity, **they can help you to build up a certain tolerance.**

As for bad surprises, they unfortunately stem from the most suspect carbohydrates because of their bad indexes, which we will discuss. But first let us talk about French fries. We see that among all methods of preparation of this tuber, frying results not only in one of the highest glycemic indexes (95), but also the highest pure carbohydrate concentration: 33g per 3.5 oz.; 5.5 times that of cooked carrots, but also 3.5 times that of potatoes boiled unpeeled. Chips are even worse than fries because their pure-carbohydrate concentration is 49g per 3.5 oz. of product with, I must note, a slightly inferior glycemic index (80).

Another bad surprise (you probably guessed it) deals with sugar. Its glycemic index is high (70), and its concentration of carbohydrates is the maximum (100%), that is, three times that of French fries and 16.6 times that of carrots. It would take 6oz. of lentils to compensate for 1oz. of sugar and lower the resulting glycemic index to 50.

The last bad surprise, of course, deals with white flour which, besides its high glycemic index (70 for a baguette, 85 for a hamburger bun), has a high pure-carbohydrate concentration (58% for very white sandwich bread, 55% for a baguette, and 74% for refined semolina). This means that if you make an exception by eating white bread or anything else made with refined flour (pizza, pastries, cakes, pancakes, waffles, etc.) you will pay because if the quantities are substantial, you will have difficulty making up for it with good carbohydrates.

Let us look at an example that demonstrates how you can put this "exception management" into practice. Imagine that you make an exception by eating a sandwich made with white bread like those you find in bus stations and convenience markets along the highway, whose glycemic index is 85. To make up for 7 oz. of this product, you would theoretically have to consume 1.5lb. of lentils to lower your resulting glycemia to 53.

Under the circumstances in which you would try to manage this type of exception, you would probably not have lentils handy. On the highway, all you will have left to use for compensation is an apple. The only problem is that apples have a higher glycemic index than lentils (33 instead of 22) and that they contain fewer pure carbohydrates (12g instead of 17g). That means that in order to bring the resulting glycemia down to 57 you would theoretically have to eat more than 2lb. of apples, which would be practically impossible.

Luckily, reality is not as cruel as theory. Other circumstances can help regulate your resulting glycemia. It has been noted, for example, that if foods with a low glycemic index are consumed before those with a high glycemic index, the compensation phenomenon is much more effective.

So in the above example, it would be better to eat the apples first, two or three are enough, in order to generate a low glycemia, then to eat the white bread. The rise in your resulting glycemia will then be much less drastic.

Further studies have reinforced this finding. They show that the rise in glycemia resulting from eating a carbohydrate with a high glycemic index at the beginning of a meal was much weaker than if the bad carbohydrate were eaten at the end of the meal.

Because of this principle, we can say that an exception made at the end of a meal (cake, bread with cheese or sweets) has a lesser chance of causing a rise in the resulting glycemia. On the contrary, if you begin your meal with exceptions (potato salad, puff pastries, ravioli, crepes, etc.) the rise in your resulting glycemia will be high and rapid, and compensating for it by eating carbohydrates with a very low index will always be more difficult.

In other words, the productivity of the compensatory carbohydrates (lentils, lettuce, chickpeas, soy, beans, green vegetables, spaghetti *al dente*, apples, pears, etc.) is always more effective when these are eaten before the exception is made. One of the most important rules to apply in the management of Phase II is to anticipate the exception you will make. It is the only way to pre-organize your compensation.

It is Sunday. And the tradition of European families, especially French families, is to prepare an excellent noon meal. Imagine that in doing so, you want to serve dessert; a strawberry pie, for example. This pie represents an exception because it contains both hyper-refined flour (index 85) and sugar (index 70). But it gets worse because white flour and sugar have a high pure-carbohydrate concentration level (58% and 100%, respectively). To compensate for this exception, you will compose the rest of the meal choosing your carbohydrates (exclusively) from among those whose glycemic index is <u>very low</u>.

First, for example, you must choose an appetizer made from raw vegetables (tomatoes, cucumbers, eggplant, mushrooms, lettuce, cabbage, bean sprouts, quinoa tabboulleh, green lentil salad, etc.) which you know have a very low glycemic index. Next, the side dishes of the main course must also be chosen from among those having a very low glycemic index (broccoli, cauliflower, green beans, and especially lentils). Naturally you must also avoid eating bread, even whole grain bread, with the cheese course, if there is any, because real integral whole grain bread is still very rare, and what is normally sold may have an index slightly over 40. Even if you drink three glasses of wine with this meal that you are planning to end with an exception, your resulting glycemia will be average, or at least sufficiently modest, to ensure that you will not experience excessive insulin secretion.

But be careful! If you allow a portion of "bad" carbohydrates into your meal, that does not mean that you should simply add good carbohydrates to compensate. In effect, this is not about eating <u>more</u> to compensate for the fact that you have eaten <u>poorly</u>. If you eat two pounds of French fries, it is not reasonable to foresee eating ten pounds of lettuce beforehand in order to compensate. Because too much carbohydrates even from low GIs will be transformed into fat anyway.

You must manage your exceptions according to their pure carbohydrate concentration. As we saw previously, even if the glycemic index of cooked carrots and French fries is similar, the pure carbohydrate concentration of the fries is eight times greater. That means that if you eat fries, your portion size must always remain modest, even symbolic. You obviously will have to apply the same rule of prudence to white flour and sugar which, as we saw before, are along with fries and chips, the mega champions of bad carbohydrates because they have both a very high glycemic index and a very high pure carbohydrate concentration.

At the risk of repeating myself, remember that you must always <u>anticipate</u> your exceptions so that you can decide on the compensation beforehand. Never sit down to eat without knowing what you will be eating from beginning to end. Otherwise, if you make a huge exception it may be too late to compensate for it. It is always best to know what is in store for you at the start of the meal so that you will be able to make the best choices.

In effect, you can make your exception during the appetizer (by eating a puff pastry, for example). You can make it during the main course (by eating a boiled potato with fish). You can make it with the cheese if you decide to eat it with bread. You can also make your exception, as we saw earlier, during dessert.

You know, for example, that it is unreasonable to make an exception during the appetizer (puffed pastries or mini quiches), then to make another with the main course (mashed potatoes or polenta), finally getting to dessert and saying, "Now I have to compensate." You will not have many choices left, unless you want to end your meal by eating two pounds of lentils or ten pounds of lettuce which would be silly anyway. This is obviously not a real solution because the amount of carbohydrates that all of that would represent would still raise your glycemia.

Phase II, then, is, as you can see, a Phase of <u>liberty</u>. But not just any liberty. It is a <u>conditional liberty</u>, or better yet, a <u>monitored liberty</u>, whose principles must become a reflex to you. They must quickly become second-nature. All exceptions, then, are possible as long as they follow two principles: that they be <u>exceptional</u> and that they be <u>managed</u>, keeping in mind their two parameters: their <u>glycemic index</u> and their <u>pure carbohydrate concentration</u>. In fact, if you had to retain just one elementary principle without getting into the technical considerations that we have just seen, it could be the following: exceptions should essentially be made on carbohydrates with a weak pure carbohydrate concentration. Their glycemic potential being weak, they are always easy to compensate for.

You may be tempted to minimize the importance of your exceptions, fostering a distinction between "small" and "big" exceptions, the second being the only one deserving your attention.

In effect, you could consider drinking three glasses of wine with dinner or eating a small piece of white-bread toast small exceptions, since it is true that the negative effects of these on your weight is almost negligible. But this attitude does not come without disadvantages because you risk minimizing the so-called "small" exceptions to the point of quickly making them habitual.

And just as small streams make large rivers, several small exceptions for which you do not compensate during a meal can have the same unhealthy effects as the large exceptions.

But the worst part, without a doubt, is that by becoming a little too tolerant, we can become so lax that little by little, we forget the fundamental principles of the Method. That is why, even if you make a small exception, you first must make yourself aware of it and then systematically integrate it into a strategy of glycemic re-balancing. It is a matter of principle.

In addition, one of the major rules to follow is <u>never</u> let yourself go, even in difficult situations. It is true that the circumstances of social and professional life can trap you by serving three bad carbohydrates in one meal; for example, a puffed pastry as an appetizer, potatoes with the main course, and a cake "cemented" with flour, butter, and sugar for dessert. In critical situations like this, no one should say that since they were not given a choice, there was nothing they could do but give in. In my opinion, this is a reprehensible attitude because there is no situation for which there is absolutely no possible move to make. In every instance, no matter how desperate it seems, you can always limit the damages. If you have convictions (and having completed a good Phase I, it would be surprising if you did not), it should be easy to resist.

Look at the vegetarians around you. The have decided, for personal reasons, not to eat meat, which is very respectable. Their convictions are always strong enough that their decision never suffers from exceptions. Even if they are invited to a barbecue, they do not eat meat.

In the application of the Method, the choices never seem so mechanical because you always have certain desires. So faced with a puffed pastry, served to you without warning, you should simply look at the rest of what is there to find the foods you can eat, carefully leaving the rest in a corner of the plate. No one will force you to eat the potatoes you have left behind. It would be surprising if you did not find a little salad, or even some cheese. You could then, without too much misgiving, make an exception on the cake, which you could even "dissect" in order to eat just the "consumable" parts. Leave the meal aware that even though you avoided catastrophe, you were not able to organize a satisfying compensation. Keep this information in the back of your mind in order to be particularly vigilant in the organization of meals that follow, where even the most elementary wisdom will lead you back to Phase I.

No matter what, the real judge of the management of your diet will always remain the needle on your scale. If you gain back a little weight, it may be for two reasons: either your pancreas has not yet found its acceptable level of tolerance and is still very sensitive to even the slightest rise in glycemia, or the amount and frequency of your exceptions are too significant. You should then take the necessary measures, doubling your attention and especially going back to Phase I as often as possible.

But there is still another indicator of the success of your exception management: the state of your health. As soon as you have gone a little too far, you will notice the harmful effects on your vitality. Then you will take the measures, somewhat instinctually, needed to make the necessary corrections.

EXAMPLE OF EXCEPTION MANAGEMENT

- EXCEPTIONS ARE IN **BOLD** PRINT
- THE COMPENSATORY CARBOHYDRATES ARE IN *ITALLICS*.

- *LENTIL* salad with olive oil vinaigrette - Veal chop - **WHITE RICE** - *GREEN SALAD* - Yogurt	- *GRATED CARROTS* - Cod - *GREEN BEANS* - **CRÈME BRÛLÉE**	- *CAESAR SALAD* without croutons - Sausage - *PURÉED SPLIT PEAS* - **VANILLA BEAN ICE CREAM**
- *AL DENTE SPAGHETTI* salad - **SLICE OF PIZZA** - *GREEN SALAD* - Sugar-free applesauce	- Foie gras on **3 COCKTAIL TOASTS** - Duck - *RATATOUILLE* - *GREEN SALAD* - Cheese	- 12 oysters and **2 slices of RYE BREAD** - Marinated salmon - *GREEN SALAD* - *CHOCOLATE MOUSSE CAKE MADE WITH 70% CACAO*
- Smoked salmon - *GREEN SALAD* - Leg of lamb - *DRIED BEANS* - cheese + **2 SLICES OF BREAD**	- Vegetable soup *(LEEKS, CABBAGE, CELERY ZUCCHINI)* - Sorrel omelet - *GREEN SALAD* - **CRÈME CARAMEL**	- *GREEN SALAD* - *CHILI* con carne - **PLUM PIE**
- *LEEKS* in vinaigrette - *LENTILS* with ham - **CHOCOLATE ECLAIR**	- *SPLIT PEA SOUP* - Cooked ham - **MASHED POTATOES WITH OLIVE OIL** - *PLAIN STRAWBERRIES*	- *ARTICHOKE HEARTS* - *AL DENTE SPAGHETTI* Sauce: Cream of *SOY* or curry - **CHEESECAKE**
- *AL DENTE SPAGHETTI SALAD* - Pork chop - *GREEN LENTILS* - Cheese + **2 SLICES OF BREAD**	- **CANTALOUPE** - **BUCKWHEAT CREPE** with eggs and ham - *GREEN SALAD* - *RASPBERRIES*	- **WATERMELON** - Rib steak - *BROCCOLI* - *FRESH POACHED APRICOTS IN FRUCTOSE*

AVERAGE PURE-CARBOHYDRATE CONCENTRATION
FOR 100 G (3.5 oz.) OF FOOD, AND G.I.

	PURE CARBOHYDRATES	GLYCEMIC INDEX
Beer	5g	110
Baked potatoes	25g	95
French fries	33g	95
Puffed rice	85g	95
Mashed potatoes	14g	90
Instant rice	24g	90
Honey	80g	90
Cooked carrots	6g	85
Corn flakes	85g	85
Plain popcorn	63g	85
T 45 flour (white bread)	58g	85
Rice cakes	24g	85
Potato chips	49g	80
Cooked broad beans	7g	80
Tapioca	94g	80
Crackers	60g	80
Pumpkin/squash	7g	75
T 55 flour (baguette)	55g	75
Watermelon	7g	75
Sweetened cereals	80g	70
Chocolate bars	60g	70
Boiled peeled potatoes	20g	70
Sugar (saccharose)	100g	70
Turnips	3g	70
Corn	22g	70
Instant non-sticky rice	24g	70
Cola	11g	70
Noodles, ravioli	23g	70
Unpeeled boiled potatoes	14g	65
Refined semolina	25g	65
Classic preserves	70g	65
Cantaloupe	6g	65
Banana	20g	65
Processed orange juice	11g	65
Raisins	66g	65
Long grain white rice	23g	60
B flour shortbread cookies	68g	55
Butter cookies	75g	55
White pasta	23g	55
Whole wheat bread (T 150)	47g	50
Buckwheat flour	65g	50
Buckwheat pancake	25g	50
Sweet potato	20g	50
Kiwi	12g	50
Basmati rice	23g	50
Whole brown rice	23g	50
Sorbet	30g	50
Whole wheat pasta (T150)	19g	45
Bran bread	40g	45
Al dente spaghetti	25g	45
Pumpernickel bread	45g	40

	PURE CARBOHYDRATES	GLYCEMIC INDEX
Fresh peas	10g	40
Grapes	16g	40
Fresh-squeezed orange juice	10g	40
Natural apple juice	17g	40
Whole rye bread	49g	40
Integral whole wheat pasta (T 200)	17g	40
Kidney beans	11g	40
Fresh integral whole wheat bread (T 200)	45g	40
Vanilla bean ice cream	25g	35
Chinese vermicelle	15g	35
Ancestral Indian corn	21g	35
Quinoa (cooked)	18g	35
Dried peas (cooked)	18g	35
Raw carrots	7g	35
Whole yogurt	4.5g	35
Low-fat yogurt	5.3g	35
Oranges	9g	35
Pears, figs	12g	35
Dried apricots	63g	35
2% milk	5g	30
All-Bran	46g	30
Peaches	9g	30
Apples	12g	30
White beans	17g	30
Green beans	3g	30
Brown lentils	17g	30
Chickpeas (cooked)	22g	30
Sugar-free marmalade	37g	30
Dark chocolate (>70% cacao)	32g	22
Green lentils	17g	22
Split peas	22g	22
Cherries	17g	22
Plums, grapefruit	10g	22
Fructose	100g	20
Soy (cooked)	15g	20
Peanuts	9g	20
Fresh apricots	10g	20
Walnuts	5g	15
Onion	5g	10
Garlic	28g	10
Green vegetables, lettuce, mushrooms, tomatoes, eggplant, green pepper, cabbage, broccoli, etc.	3-5g	≈10

Chapter 6

HYPOGLYCEMIA
THE DISEASE OF THE CENTURY

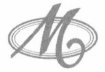

We have already learned that metabolism is the transformation of food into vital elements the body can use. For example, when we speak of the metabolism of lipids, we are referring to the transformation of fats. The main goal of this book is really to study the metabolism of carbohydrates and its consequences.

We saw in previous chapters that insulin (a hormone secreted by the pancreas) plays a determining role in the metabolism of carbohydrates. The basic function of insulin is to act upon the glucose found in the blood, making it penetrate the cells and therefore, assuring the functioning of the organs and the formation of muscular and hepatic glycogen, and sometimes stored fats. Insulin expels the glucose (sugar) from the blood and, thus, lowers the level of sugar in the blood (glycemia). If too much insulin is produced by the pancreas (if the amount of insulin is disproportionate to the glucose that it must help to metabolize), then the blood sugar level will fall to an abnormally low level. The body is then in a state of hypoglycemia.

Hypoglycemia, then, is not always caused by a sugar deficiency, but often by an excessive secretion of insulin (hyperinsulinism) following an abuse of carbohydrates with a high glycemic index (potatoes, white bread, corn, etc.). If, for example, you suddenly feel tired around 11 o'clock in the morning, most often your blood sugar is lower than normal. You are experiencing hypoglycemia. If you eat a bad carbohydrate (high GI), like a cookie or some other sweet, your body will rapidly transform it into glucose. The presence of glucose in the blood will make your sugar level go up, and you will definitely feel better. But the presence of glucose in the blood will automatically trigger a secretion of insulin that will cause the glucose to disappear and will reestablish your hypoglycemia with a sugar level that is even lower than that with which you started. It is this vicious circle that can lead to addictive behavior.

A number of scientists have considered alcoholism a consequence of chronic hypoglycemia. As soon as an alcoholic's blood alcohol level begins to drop, he or she feels down and needs a drink. But since he or she usually also consumes carbohydrates with very high glycemic levels, the alcohol increases the risk of hypoglycemia, provoking supplementary fatigue. The alcoholic will gladly relieve this new drop in energy by consuming yet another alcoholic drink, giving him or her an illusory and transitional feeling of elation. We then understand that the risk of hypoglycemia is made even greater when alcoholic beverages are sweet themselves (beer, gin and tonic, whiskey and Coke, screwdriver, sangria, port wine, etc.).

Adolescents, large consumers of highly sweetened beverages, have a saw-tooth-shaped glycemic curve much like that of alcoholics. Some American doctors have claimed that this situation actually predisposes young people to alcoholism, which is raging more and more rampantly on college campuses. Adolescents' bodies are in some ways prepared, almost conditioned, to move from soda to alcohol. This is just one more reason to make parents aware of the potential risk of abusing certain bad carbohydrates.

The symptoms of hypoglycemia are the following:
- fatigue, sudden exhaustion
- irritability
- nervousness
- aggressiveness
- impatience
- anxiety
- yawning, lack of concentration
- headaches
- excessive perspiration
- sweaty palms
- lack of professional efficiency
- digestive problems
- nausea
- difficulty of expression

The list is not long, yet it is impressive. This does not mean that one who suffers from hypoglycemia will have all these symptoms, nor does it mean that the symptoms that do appear will be permanent. Some, in fact, will be quite ephemeral and could disappear as soon as you eat.

You may have noticed that some people become progressively nervous, unstable, and even aggressive, as the time that they normally eat approaches. Among these symptoms, one occurs more frequently than the others do. You have probably noticed it yourselves. It is **fatigue**.

Fatigue is one of the characteristics of our era. The more people sleep, have time for leisure, and go on vacation, the more tired they are. When they get up in the morning, they are already "beat". By the end of the morning, they are not going to make it. In the beginning of the afternoon they are sleeping on their desks – this is the sudden after-lunch slump. At the end of the afternoon, it is all they can do to pick up their things and go home. They are dragging. In the evening, they do nothing but doze in front of the television. Once they go to bed, they are no longer tired. When they finally do find sleep, it is already time to get up, and a new cycle begins. So we blame the stress of modern life, noise, transportation, pollution, lack of magnesium, etc.

All we know how to do to fight this phenomenon is drink a cup of strong coffee, take vitamin and mineral supplements, or do yoga. Most of the time, fatigue is a problem stemming from glycemia and nutritional unbalance.

The amount of sugar in the blood (glycemia) of our contemporaries is chronically and abnormally low. This situation is the consequence of a diet containing excessive amounts of carbohydrates, especially those having a high glycemic index – too much sugar, too many sweetened beverages, too much white bread, too many potatoes, white rice, and cookies that cause an excessive secretion of insulin.

For a long time we believed that only people who could easily gain weight could be hypoglycemic. Recent studies done in the United States in the last ten years have shown that many thin people are also victims of hypoglycemia because of their excessive consumption of sugar and carbohydrates with a high glycemic index. The difference between them is their metabolism. Some gain weight, the others do not. But as far as blood sugar is concerned, the phenomenon and its consequences are the same.

These studies also reveal that women are more sensitive to glycemic variations. This could explain some women's frequent mood changes. In any case, it is proven that postpartum depression is a direct consequence of a state of hypoglycemia linked to birth.

If you seriously put the Method I have taught you into practice, you will quickly notice that besides weight loss, there will be other positive effects. **You will rediscover the joy of living, optimism, and vitality.** If you were experiencing "slumps" you will not have them anymore. You will experience physical and mental renewal.

When you eliminate sugar from your diet and limit your intake of bad carbohydrates, your pancreas will stop secreting excessive amounts of insulin, and the amount of sugar in your blood will stabilize itself at its ideal level. "Good carbohydrates" (those that have a low glycemic index) do not cause reactionary hypoglycemia.

According to the scientists and doctors with whom I work, hypoglycemia is one of the most difficult diseases to diagnose. The symptoms are so numerous and varied that general practitioners practically never acknowledge it. One of the reasons may be that little information about it is made available to medical students. Very few class hours are actually devoted to the topic.

The best way to know if you are hypoglycemic is to put the nutritional rules provided in the previous chapters into practice. Less than a week after beginning, you will happily notice a phenomenal increase in your well-being.

Much unexplainable fatigue originates from a vitamin, mineral, or other nutritional deficiency. Those who follow low-calorie diets lack important nutrients because they do not eat enough. The phenomenon is accentuated by the fact that overworked soil has become poor, and the vegetation from which it grows contains fewer of these nutrients.

To stay healthy and avoid hypoglycemia, you must eat carbohydrates that have a low glycemic index (fruits, whole grain products, dried beans, green vegetables, etc.). When possible, you should eat them raw. That way you are sure to obtain the correct ration of nutrients needed for optimal functioning of the body.

Chapter 7

VITAMINS, MINERALS AND TRACE ELEMENTS

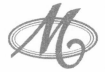

Our modern diet lacks vitamins, minerals and trace elements. Not only have refining techniques eliminated them, but also most industrial processing, whether at the production stage or the conservation stage, tends to considerably diminish them, as do the sometimes-hazardous cooking methods. For the most part, we have been aware of the consequences of their complete absence for a long time. Every day we discover more harmful effects of vitamin, mineral, and trace element deficiencies. Among the most evident are fatigue and difficulty with weight loss.

VITAMINS

The word vitamin inevitably evokes vitality. It is important to note that no chemical reactions in the body would be possible without vitamins. They intervene in the functioning of hundreds of enzymes by triggering biochemical reactions within our body's cells.

Living in Western countries where there is an abundance of food, we should never lack vitamins. Yet this is exactly what is currently happening to much of the population. Besides the followers of low-calorie diets who are not getting the nutritional balance they need from their food, the rest of the population also lacks that balance because of poor eating habits.

Everyone knows that fruits and fiber-rich foods contain a significant concentration of vitamins. According to statistics taken by Professor Cloarec, 37% of French people never eat fruit, and 32% never eat green vegetables. We also know that in other countries (especially Anglo-Saxon countries), fruit and vegetable consumption is even lower than that.

This situation is worsened by the fact that the people of those same countries mainly base their diets on refined foods whose vitamins have been removed, like white flour, white rice, etc. Nevertheless, vitamins are indispensable to the functioning of the body, in which they react in infinitesimal quantities. Since the body is incapable of synthesizing them, that is, of making them itself, it must get them from our daily food intake.

We distinguish:
- water-soluble (or hydrosoluble) vitamins that are not able to be stored within the body. These are the vitamins B, C, and PP that we often lose in cooking water, which is no longer kept for making soup as it used to be.
- fat-soluble (or liposoluble) vitamins that can be stored within the body. Among them are vitamins A, D, E, and K.

VITAMIN DEFICIENCY

After World War II, the sociological transformation of Western societies and the increase in population resulted into two phenomena: urbanization and desertion of rural areas. It not only became necessary to produce more, it also became necessary to produce differently because, for the first time in the history of humanity, the places where food was consumed and the places where it was produced were different.

In order to increase output, agriculture quickly developed the use of chemical fertilizers, pesticides, insecticides, herbicides, and fungicides. As a solution to the problem of the time it took for food to be transported to the places it was consumed, new conservation techniques were created, rendering the use of additives and chemical preservatives commonplace.

These changes ultimately led to a degeneration of soil and a surcharge of undesirable chemical substances in produce. In this way, fruits, vegetables, and grains have lost considerable amounts of vitamins and even minerals and trace elements. It explains why the amount of vitamins A, B1, B2, B3 and C has diminished by more than 30% in certain vegetables, depending on how they are grown. Vitamin E, for example, has practically disappeared in lettuce, peas, apples, and parsley, in much the same way that vitamin PP has vanished from strawberries. From one bunch of spinach to another, you may find anywhere from 3 to 150 mg of total vitamins for 100g of product.

The prevailing taste for white bread throughout the nineteenth century encouraged research in flour-refining processes. The 1875, discovery of the cylinder-run mill tolled the nutritional bell for bread. Because of systematic industrial refining, bread was stripped of most of its nutritional substance: fiber, protein, essential fatty acids, vitamins, minerals, and trace elements. Stripped of all its vital ingredients through persistent beating, wheat grain is nothing more than almost pure starch, whose benefit to the body is solely energetic.

Inversely, we can raise the vitamin content of certain foods by, for example, germinating the seeds. But this is only vigorously practiced in areas that are still quite isolated and inhabited by very health-conscious people, like followers of organic agriculture.

THE ALTERATION OF VITAMINS BY COOKING

Excessively long storage, exposure to air, and cooking can lead to a great loss of vitamin C in fruits and vegetables. The greatest losses occur when food is cooked for a very long time. Thus, a short cooking time at a low temperature only leads to a small vitamin loss. Keep this in mind when eating dishes like stew, which are cooked for hours.

LACK OF VITAMINS FROM DIETARY DEFICIENCY

If you eat an insufficient amount of food, which is inevitably the case when following low-calorie diets, you create a vitamin deficiency.

HOW DO YOU AVOID VITAMIN LOSS?

- Use fresh products instead of foods that have already been stocked for several days.

LOW (1500) CALORIE DIET	
VITAMINS	% DAILY VALUE OBTAINED
A	30
E	60
B1	40
B2	48
B6	49
C	45
PP	43
B5	40
B9	38

VITAMIN	SOURCES	SIGNS OF DEFICIENCY
A (retinol)	liver, egg yolks, milk, butter, carrots, spinach, tomatoes, apricots	Difficulty with night vision Sensitivity to reverberation Dry skin Easily sunburned skin Ear, nose and throat infections
Provitamin A (betacarotene)	carrots, watercress, spinach, mango, cantaloupe, apricots, broccoli, peaches, butter	
D (calciferol)	liver, tuna, sardines, egg yolks, mushrooms, butter, cheese, the sun	Children: rickets Elderly: osteoporosis, bone demineralization
E (tocopherol)	oils, hazlenuts, almonds, whole grains, milk, butter, eggs, dark chocolate, whole wheat bread	Muscular fatigue, cardio vasuclar risk, skin aging
K	Made by bacteria in colon. liver, cabbage, spinach, eggs, broccoli, meat, cauliflower	Hemorrhaging
B1 (thiamin)	yeast, wheat germ, pork, giblets, fish, whole grains, whole wheat bread	Fatigue, irritability, difficulty with memory, lack of appetite, depression, muscular weakness
B2 (riboflavin)	yeast, liver, kidneys, cheese, almonds, eggs, fish, milk, cacao	Seborrheic dermatitis, reddish rash, light sensitivity, fragile or dull hair, lesions on lips and tongue
PP or vitamin B3 or niacin or nicotimic acid	yeast, wheat bran, liver, meat, kidneys, fish, whole wheat bread, dates, legumes, intestinal flora	Fatigue, insomnia, anorexia, depression, lesions of the skin & mucous membranes

VITAMIN	SOURCES	SIGNS OF DEFICIENCY
B5 (pantothenic acid)	yeast, liver, kidneys, eggs, meat, mushrooms, grains, leguminous fruits	Fatigue, headache, nausea, vomiting, moodiness, orthostatic hypertension, hair loss
B6 (pyridoxine)	yeast, wheat germ, soy, liver, kidneys, meat, fish, brown rice, avocados, legumes, whole wheat bread	Fatigue, depression, irritability, vertigo, nausea, skin lesions, sugar cravings, headaches from glutamate
B8 (or biotin or vitamin H)	intestinal flora, yeast, liver, kidneys, chocolate, eggs, mushrooms, chicken, cauliflower, legumes, meat, whole wheat bread	Fatigue, loss of appetite, nausea, muscular fatigue, oily skin, hair loss, insomnia, depression, neurological problems
B9 (folic acid)	yeast, liver, oysters, soy, spinach, watercress, green vegetables, legumes, whole wheat bread, cheese, milk, wheat germ	Fatigue, memory loss, insomnia, depression, mental confusion, difficulty scarring, neurological problems
B12 (cyanobalamin)	liver, kidneys, oysters, herring, fish, meat, eggs	Fatigue, irritability, palor, anemia, loss of appetite, difficulty sleeping, neuromuscular pain, memory loss, depression
C (asorbic acid)	rose petals, black currants, parsley, kiwi, broccoli, green vegetables, citrus fruits, liver, kidneys	Fatigue, drowsiness, loss of appetite, muscular pain, weak resistance to infection, frequent breathlessness

- If possible, buy your vegetables on a daily basis, as you need them, from a farmer's market or a local truck farmer.
- Use as little water as possible in preparation (washing, soaking).
- Opt for raw fruits and vegetables (except in cases of digestive intolerance).
- Peel and grate as little as possible.
- Avoid cooking for long periods of time at high temperatures.
- Cook at a low temperature; in particular, lightly steam vegetables.
- Avoid keeping foods hot for prolonged periods of time.
- Keep your cooking water to make soup; it contains hydrosoluble vitamins.
- Try to avoid having leftovers, which get put in the refrigerator and reheated.
- Reduce quantity, but choose quality by favoring, for example, organic produce; the cost is about the same.
- Roasting and grilling help to conserve the vitamins in meats.
- Frozen products are richer in vitamins than canned goods.
- Do not expose milk to light.

MINERALS AND TRACE ELEMENTS

Many chemical reactions take place in the human body. These different reactions could not occur without the presence of minerals and trace elements, which act indirectly by way of enzymes. For example, there could be no transmission of nerve impulses without sodium or potassium. There would be no muscular activity without calcium, and no thyroid hormones without iodine. In the same way, there would be no blood oxygenation without iron, nor would there be correct assimilation of glucose without chromium.

Among these micronutrients, we distinguish:
- Minerals like calcium, phosphorus, potassium, sodium, sulfur, and magnesium.
- Trace elements like chromium, cobalt, zinc, copper and selenium, which function in infinitesimal quantities.

A lack of minerals and trace elements can be harmful. In effect, we know that:
- a manganese deficit encourages hyperglycemia, and
- a nickel, chromium and zinc deficit contributes to insulin resistance.

Are supplements a good solution?

It is impossible to imagine that a deficit in micronutrients linked to poor eating habits could easily be fixed by supplements in the form of tablets or capsules. These synthetic products, even if they can help with serious deficiencies, are <u>not easily absorbed</u> by the intestines.

Thus, it is better to pursue a normal diet, varying in its quantities of minerals and trace elements needed by the body. That is why I encourage the consumption of fruits, vegetables, salads, legumes, and whole grains.

The only supplements I can support are beer yeast and wheat germ, two natural products that contain many of the nutrients our modern diet is so seriously lacking. What is more, beer yeast is rich in chromium, which helps increase the body's tolerance for glucose, therefore leading to a lowering of glycemia and insulinemia. <u>Thus it indirectly helps you to lose weight!</u>

You can add one teaspoon of beer yeast or wheat germ, alternating every other day, to a dairy product eaten at breakfast.

FOR 100 G (3.5 oz.)	BEER YEAST	WHEAT GERM
Water	6 g	11 g
Proteins	42 g	26 g
Carbohydrates	19 g	34 g
Lipids	2 g	10 g
Fiber	22 g	17 g
Potassium	1 800 mg	850 mg
Magnesium	230 mg	260 mg
Phosphorus	1 700 mg	1 100 mg
Calcium	100 mg	70 mg
Iron	18 mg	9 mg
Beta Carotene	0.01 mg	0 mg
Vitamin B1	10 mg	2 mg
Vitamin B2	5 mg	0.7 mg
Vitamin B5	12 mg	1.7 mg
Vitamin B6	4 mg	3 mg
Vitamin B12	0.01 mg	0 mg
Folic acid	4 mg	430 mg
Vitamin PP	46 mg	4.5 mg
Vitamin E	0 mg	21 mg

Chapter 8

HYPERCHOLESTEROLEMIA, CARDIOVASCULAR DISEASE AND DIETARY HABITS

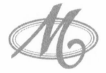

According to the expression of a doctor, "AIDS kills little but with much ado, while cardio-vascular diseases kill every second but in silence!"

An American dies every 90 seconds of a heart attack! Cardiovascular ailments remain, in effect, and by far, the main cause of death (close to 40% in France, in front of cancer, which represents about a quarter of deaths).

Huge informational efforts have been made these last two decades in all western countries, and particularly in the United States, to achieve better prevention. But the fight is far from being won because the frequency of cardio-vascular illnesses is inversely proportional to that of the level of education, of family revenue, and of the degree of job qualification.

Thus, it is in underprivileged areas, which are the most affected, that the birth rates are higher. That is why there is every reason to fear a rise in the number of deaths by cardio-vascular disease in the 21st century, despite the active prevention campaigns.

Yet the risk factors of cardio-vascular disease are well-known. These are LDL cholesterol, triglycerides, arterial hypertension, diabetes, obesity, but also smoking, lack of exercise, and stress. These normally take 30 to 40 years to manifest themselves and become vital threats, but forms exist where heredity can make the prognosis worse. That is why nearly 5% of those dying from cardio-vascular illnesses are younger than 25.

In the previous chapters, we discovered that it is the consumption of high-glycemic carbohydrates that is the principal responsible for weight gain. This does not necessarily mean, as we have so often restated, that you can eat fat *ad libitum* because too much could, in effect, compromise your general health.

We also heavily insisted on the fact that it was good to make wise choices from among fats because some could increase cardio-vascular risks while others had, on the contrary, the advantage of making up a factor of prevention.

But before returning to a more detailed study of the properties of fat according to the nature of their fatty acids, it is beneficial to have an understanding of cholesterol.

CHOLESTEROL: A FALSELY ACCUSED INTRUDER

Cholesterol is not an intruder. The substance is even indispensable to the formation of certain hormones. The body contains around 100g of it, divided among the tissues of the nervous system, the nerves, and the different cells.

The body makes much of its own cholesterol (up to 70%); bile, in particular, releases 800 to 1200 mg per day into the small intestine. Only 30% of your body's cholesterol comes from your food; therefore, the amount of cholesterol in your blood is only slightly dependent upon the amount of cholesterol contained in food. Rather, your blood cholesterol level is linked to the type of fatty acids you eat (saturated, mono or polyunsaturated).

THE GOOD AND THE BAD

Cholesterol is not isolated in the blood because it is attached to proteins. There are two categories of these proteins. Low Density Lipoproteins, or LDLs, distribute cholesterol to the cells, especially the cells of the artery walls, where fatty deposits form. LDL cholesterol was christened "bad cholesterol" because in the long run it clogs the interior of these vessels.

This artery obstruction can cause cardiovascular problems:
- angina pectoris or a myocardial infarction
- arteritis in the lower limbs
- a stroke, which could eventually lead to paralysis

High Density Lipoproteins, or HDLs, guide cholesterol to the liver for elimination. HDL cholesterol was labeled "good cholesterol" because it does not cause vascular deposits. On the contrary, it cleans the arteries of their atheromatic deposits. We know that the higher the HDL level, the lesser the risk of cardiovascular problems.

BLOOD CHOLESTEROL LEVEL

Today's norms are much stricter than those that were prevalent for many years. Three specific notions must be retained:
- Total cholesterol (HDL+LDL) must be less than or equal to two grams per quart of blood,
- LDL cholesterol must be less than 1.30 grams per quart of blood,
- HDL cholesterol must be greater than 0.45 grams per quart of blood for men and 0.55 grams per quart for women.

CARDIOVASCULAR RISKS

Cardiovascular risk is doubled if your total cholesterol level reaches 2.2 grams per quart of blood, and by four if it is greater than 2.60 grams per quart. Yet it has been observed that 15% of infarctions occurred in subjects whose percentage of total cholesterol was less than two grams per quart. For that reason, this notion has no completely relative significance.

What is more significant is the total amount of LDL and HDL in the blood, and most importantly, the rapport between total cholesterol and HDL, which must be less than 4.5. Knowing that lowering your cholesterol by 12.5% (if your numbers are critical) lowers your risk of myocardial infarction by 19%, you ought to take this subject very seriously.

Yet cholesterol, even if it is the most talked about risk factor in cardiovascular disease (especially in the media), is not the only one. Many other factors, which we can deal with by our food choices, can cause vascular alteration: hyperglycemia (with or without diabetes), hyperinsulinism, hypertriglyceridemia, antioxidant deficiency (vitamins A, C, and E, beta carotene, zinc, copper, selenium, and **polyphenols**), not forgetting tobacco products.

NUTRITIONAL TREATMENT

Doctors will be able to prescribe certain medications for cases of hypercholesterolemia, but this should always be a last resort. In most cases, good dietary management is enough. Here is some advice you can follow, both to lower your cholesterol if it is too high, and to prevent cardiovascular risk in general.

1. Lose weight.

It has been shown that in most cases weight loss leads to improvement in all biological aspects. A lower cholesterol level is certainly the one that will appear the most rapidly, as long as you do not make the mistake of consuming too many bad lipids (saturated fats).

2. Is it necessary to limit cholesterol intake?

Food contains a variable level of cholesterol. Egg yolks, giblets, and coconut all contain a lot of cholesterol. For a long time, the World Health Organization has been advising that the recommended daily intake of 300 mg not be exceeded.

Nevertheless, recent work has shown this dietetic advice to be rather secondary. A daily intake of 1000 mg of cholesterol only leads to about a 5% rise in cholesterolemia. So you can overlook the cholesterol content of food. On the other hand, you must keep in mind the amount of saturated fats you consume.

3. Choose your lipids wisely.

In Chapter 2 we saw, under the classification of foods, that fats should be divided into three categories:

SATURATED FATS, found especially in meats, very fatty pork products, eggs, milk, whole dairy products, cheese, and palm oil. These fats raise your total cholesterol level, especially LDL cholesterol, which deposits itself on the artery walls, thus fostering vascular problems. Recent publications show that eggs and fermented cheeses have a much smaller effect on cholesterol than what we once thought. As for poultry, if the skin is removed, it contains very little saturated fat. Eating poultry, then, has very little effect on your cholesterol level.

	Lipids for 100 g	Saturated fats
Andouilles*	8 g	3.2 g
Lean cooked ham*	3 g	1.1 g
Smoked ham*	13 g	1.7 g
Head cheese*	13 g	4.6 g
Foie gras**	45 g	17 g
Dry sausage**	30 g	12.1 g
Bacon**	31 g	11.1 g
Black pudding**	34 g	12.6 g
Mortadella	30 g	12.4 g
Pork liver paté**	37 g	15 g
Salami**	42 g	16.4 g
Saveloy**	28 g	11 g
Frankfurters**	24 g	10 g
Garlic sausage*	28 g	10.70 g

*Meats with little fat
**Very fatty meats. To be avoided or only very moderately consumed

POLYUNSATURATED ANIMAL FATS. These are essentially the fatty acids contained in fish fats.

For a long time, it was thought that Eskimos, who have a diet composed 98% of fish fats, did not experience cardiovascular problems for genetic reasons. It was later recognized that, in fact, the kinds of foods they ate made up the best recipe for prevention. Eating fish fats leads to a significant lowering of triglycerides and prevents thrombosis. It has also been found that, contrary to what was once believed, the fattier the fish, the greater its cardiovascular benefits. So I encourage you to eat salmon, tuna, sardines, mackerel, anchovies, and herring.

POLYUNSATURATED VEGETABLE FATS. The main one is linoleic acid, found especially in sunflower, corn, soy and peanut oils. Linoleic acid is especially present in nut, soy, and rapeseed oils.

Polyunsaturated fatty acids are also found in oleaginous fruits: walnuts, almonds, peanuts, and sesame seeds. The problem with polyunsaturated fatty acids is that they oxidize very easily.

Oxidation especially occurs when the body lacks antioxidants. Thus, polyunsaturated vegetable fats can be as atherogenic (causing atherosclerosis) as saturated fatty acids.

UNSATURATED "TRANS" FATTY ACIDS. These are fatty acids that can appear after the industrial processing of mono- or polyunsaturated fatty acids: margarine, industrial bread, cookies, pastries, candy, and instant meals. These "trans" fatty acids are very atherogenic and just as dangerous as saturated fats. That is why it is better to use natural products as often as possible, prepared at home, rather than to call on industrial ready-made products.

MONOUNSATURATED FATTY ACIDS. The main one is oleic acid, which is especially found in olive oil.

Olive oil could be considered the champion of fats having a positive effect on cholesterol. In effect, it is the only one able to lower bad cholesterol (LDL) and raise good cholesterol (HDL).

Having heard this, some of you will have recognized that eating tuna in olive oil can be your passport against circulatory problems. But olive oil is not the only product containing monounsaturated fatty acids. It is also present in poultry (goose and duck fat) and foie gras.

4. Choose your carbohydrates wisely.

Hyperglycemia and hyperinsulinism are authentic factors in cardiovascular risk (mainly arterial hypertension and hypertriglyceridemia. That is why a too-frequent consumption of carbohydrates with a high glycemic index (potatoes, white flour and sugar) must be avoided by choosing carbohydrates having a very low glycemic index (lentils, peas, chickpeas, fruit, green vegetables and whole grain cereals). In cases of hypertriglyceridemia, it is also imperative to avoid the consumption of bad carbohydrates and/or limit alcohol.

5. Eat more fiber.

The presence of fiber in the digestive tract improves the effect of lipids' metabolism. It has also been noted that the consumption of pectin (by eating apples) leads to a slight drop in cholesterol level, which is also true of all other soluble fiber, contained in oats and legumes (white beans and lentils).

FOODS RICH IN ANTI-OXYDANTS

Vitamin E	Vitamin C	Betacarotene	Copper
wheat germ oil	rose petals	raw carrots	oysters
corn oil	black currants	watercress	veal liver
soy oil	parsley	spinach	mutton liver
sunflower oil	kiwi	mango	muscles
peanut oil	broccoli	cantaloupe	cocoa powder
rapeseed oil	sorrel	apricots	beef liver
olive oil	raw green peppers	broccoli	wheat germ
wheat germ	tarragon	peaches	white beans
hazlenuts, almonds	raw white cabbage	tomatoes	hazlenuts
germed grains	watercress	oranges	dried peas
walnuts, peanuts	raw red cabbage	dandelion	oatmeal
wild rice	lemon, orange	chevril, parsley	walnuts
			cervelle

Vitamin A	Selenium	Zinc	Plyphenols
codliver oil	oysters	oysters	wine
liver	chicken liver	dried peas	grape seeds
butter	beef liver	duck liver	green tea
cooked eggs	fish	beer yeast	olive oil
fresh apricots	eggs	dried beans	onions
cheese	mushrooms	kidneys	apples
salmon	onions	eel	
whole milk	whole wheat bread	lentils	
sardines	brown rice	meat	
sour cream	lentils	whole wheat bread	
	cervelle		

6. Take in plenty of antioxidants.

In the body, certain metabolic reactions can lead to a oxidation phenomena called free radicals, which are also the consequence of the hazardous effects of the environment (smoking and pollution) and even exercise that is too intense. Free radicals alter the cells and cause lesions on blood vessels. They also accelerate the aging process and cause many types of cancer.

To fight against free radicals, you should consume sufficient amounts of antioxidants: vitamin A (and especially its precursor, beta-carotene), vitamin C, vitamin E, selenium, zinc, copper, and **polyphenols** which we mainly find in red wine.

7. You can drink wine.

Studies by Professors Masquelier and Renaud have shown that consuming one to three glasses of wine (especially red) per day reduces cardiovascular risk. In effect, wine contains substances that lower LDL cholesterol (bad cholesterol) and raise HDL cholesterol (good cholesterol). It protects the artery walls and makes the blood flow more easily, preventing thrombosis.

8. Improve the hygiene of your life.

Stress, smoking, and lack of exercise also have a negative effect on cholesterol. Better health depends not only on the cure, but also on prevention.

SUMMARY OF MEASURES TO TAKE FOR THOSE WITH HYPERCHOLESTEROLEMIA

OR WHO SIMPLY WANT TO PREVENT CARDIOVASCULAR RISK.
- Lose weight if you are obese.
- Lower your meat consumption.

- Choose low fat meats (lean beef).
- Replace meats as often as possible with poultry (skinless).
- Avoid fatty pork products and giblets.
- Opt for fish.
- Eat only small amounts of butter and margarine (max. 1 tbsp. per day).
- Reduce your cheese consumption.
- Drink skim milk and eat fat free dairy products.
- Limit your consumption of carbohydrates with a high glycemic index (potatoes, white flour and sugar).
- Increase your consumption of carbohydrates with a very low glycemic index that also contain fiber (fruit, whole grains, vegetables and legumes).
- Increase your consumption of mono- and polyunsaturated vegetable oils (olive, sunflower and rapeseed).
- Commit to getting enough antioxidants and chromium (**beer yeast and wheat germ**).
- If you wish, drink red wine, rich in tannin (2-4 glasses per day).
- Control your stress.
- Exercise regularly (walk, swim, bike, ride a horse or play tennis).
- Quit smoking.

Chapter 9

SUGAR IS POISON

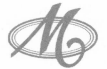

Sugar is poison.   The damage it has done to 20th century society is as serious as the effects of alcohol and tobacco put together. Everyone knows it. All the doctors in the world say so. There is not a colloquium of pediatricians, cardiologists, psychiatrists and dentists that does not mention the dangers of sugar, particularly the dangers of the exponentially rising consumption of it.

In ancient times sugar, as it is used today, practically did not exist. The Greeks did not even have a word for it. Around 325 BC, Alexander the Great, who had pushed his world conquest to the plains of the Indus, described sugar as "a sort of honey found in canes and reeds growing at the water's edge." In the first century AD, Pliny the Elder also referred to it as the "honey of the cane." It was not until the time of Nero that the word **saccharum** was created to designate this exotic product.

It was in the seventh century AD that the cultivation of sugar cane began to appear in Persia and Sicily. Little by little, the Arab countries also acquired a taste for it. In 1953, a German scholar, Dr. Rauwolf, noted in his journal that "the Turks and the Moors are no longer the intrepid soldiers they had been before they discovered sugar."

Sugar cane was discovered in the West during the Crusades. Soon after, the Spanish tried to cultivate it in the south of their country. Sugar commerce became an economic stake with the conquest of the New World and the triangular trade route. Portugal, Spain, and England became rich by trading this raw material for slaves, whose work contributed to the development of sugar cane cultivation. By 1700, France already had a number of refineries.

The defeat of Napoleon at the Battle of Trafalgar in 1805 and the continental blockade that resulted led him, against scientists' recommendations, to look for a way to produce sugar from beets. This only became truly possible after the 1812 discovery of the extraction procedure by Benjamin Delessert. Several dozen years later there was already a surplus of sugar in France, but its consumption had still not developed into what it is today.

In 1880 the rate of sugar consumption was around 17 pounds[17] per person per year, which is about five sugar cubes per day. Twenty years later, in 1900, it had more than doubled, having reached 37 pounds. In 1960 Europeans were consuming 66 pounds, and in 1972, 83 pounds. In just two centuries, the average European consumption of sugar has gone from less than two pounds to almost 83.

In three million years, humans have never so abruptly and brutally altered their eating habits in such a short period of time.

---

[17] In 1789, about a hundred years earlier, the consumption rate was still less than two pounds per year per person.

And still the Europeans are far from being the worst off in this category. North American countries have a more serious situation because their sugar consumption, particularly in the United States, is around 130 pounds per person per year. According to the most recent statistics, this sugar consumption is, despite the warning signals, still growing.

What is most worrisome is that the proportion of "hidden sugar"[18] is rising even more rapidly. In 1970 the amount of sugar indirectly absorbed (through beverages, sweets, preserves, etc.) was 58% of total sugar consumption. By 1980 it had risen above 65%. This hidden sugar can be misleading. With the introduction of artificial sweeteners and the firm recommendations of the medical world, the direct consumption of sugar (cubes or granulated) is stagnating, and even dropping.

On the other hand, the indirect consumption of sugar is alarming. It is especially rampant among children and adolescents. A two-liter bottle of cola contains the equivalent of about 46 sugar cubes. The extra-sweet taste is concealed by the coldness of the drink.

The urge to drink sweet beverages (soft drinks) is now completely integrated into our eating habits. The companies that manufacture them are powerful international corporations, and the impact of their advertising is absolutely phenomenal. It is frightening to see how they have been able to set up in third-world countries where the population's dietary needs are sometimes not even met.

The consumption of ice cream and other frozen desserts that used to be reserved for parties or special outings has now become commonplace with the widespread use of freezers. The installation of automatic candy and snack machines in all public

---

[18] "Hidden sugar" is sugar added to commercial foods and beverages.

places is also a constant appeal to consumers. Obtaining junk food is even easier and more tempting thanks to the fact that it is relatively inexpensive. In supermarkets, a pound of candy costs less than a dollar. The potential consumer is constantly and permanently tempted. Resisting these goodies becomes an act of heroism.

It is stating the obvious to say that sugar is responsible for a great number of health problems. Everyone seems to know it, but that will not convince us to change our eating habits or, even less, those of our children. Excessive sugar consumption (like that of any food having a high glycemic index) can cause an increase in cardiovascular risk, especially because of the hazardous effects of hyperglycemia, hyperinsulinism, and hypertriglyceridemia.[19] Dr. Yudkin cites the East African tribes Mascar and Samburee, whose diets, very high in fat, are almost completely devoid of sugar. The incidence of coronary disease in these tribes is almost nonexistent. On the other hand, the residents of St. Helena Island, who eat lots of sugar and very little fat, have suffered a great number of coronary illnesses.

Cavities, linked to excessive sugar consumption, are so widespread in Western countries that the World Health Organization ranks dental and oral diseases third, after cardiovascular diseases and cancer, among the top health problems afflicting industrialized countries.

When associating sugar with illness, we naturally think of diabetes. But we are wrong to believe that diabetes only affects those prone to it through heredity. Not all adult diabetics are obese, but most are. Unfortunately the United States has one of

---

[19] Epidemological studies done for twelve years by Professor W. Willett of Harvard's School of Public Health have clearly shown the responsibility of sugar in the prevalence of obesity and diabetes in the US. In addition, according to Dr. Edward Giovannucci, also of Harvard University, 23 epidemological studies show a correllation between excessive sugar consumption and colon cancer.

the greatest problems with obesity, which is a direct result of a diet rich in bad carbohydrates, especially sugar. Having read the previous chapters, you now understand that sugar, a purely chemical product, can cause hypoglycemia, generally upset metabolism, and provoke a number of digestive disorders.

Finally, it is important to know that sugar leads to vitamin B1 deficiencies. Large quantities of this vitamin are needed to absorb carbohydrates. Sugar, just like all refined starches (white flour, white rice, etc.), is completely devoid of vitamin B1, creating a deficit whose consequences generally include: neurasthenia (nervous exhaustion), fatigue, depression, muscle fatigue and loss of concentration, memory, and perception. This is a subject that should be studied more in depth for children experiencing difficulty in school.

ARTIFICIAL SWEETENERS

I have already advised you to eliminate sugar completely. Obviously it will be impossible to avoid hidden sugars like those in desserts, but if you are able to eliminate granulated sugar and sugar cubes, you will already be successful.

You can do one of two things – give it up or replace it with artificial sweeteners. There are four major artificial sweeteners. None of them, except polyols, contains potential energy; therefore, they have no nutritional value.

1. Saccharine

Discovered in 1879, this is the oldest sugar substitute. It is not used by the body and has a sweetening potential of more than 350 times that of the saccharose in natural sugar. It has the advantage of being very stable in acidic substances and can tolerate medium temperatures. Saccharine was the most commercialized sweetener until the discovery of aspartame.

2. Cyclamates

Even though their discovery dates back to 1937, cyclamates are not nearly as well known as saccharine. They are made for benzene, and their sweetening potential is less than that of saccharine. Some people find they leave an aftertaste. The advantage of cyclamates is that they are completely thermostable; in other words, completely resistant to high temperatures. The most commonly used cyclamate is made from sodium cyclamate. Other kinds include calcium cyclamate and cyclamate acid.

3. Aspartame

In Chicago in 1965, James Schlatter, a researcher at Searle Laboratories, discovered aspartame. This sugar substitute is a combination of two natural amino acids: aspartic acid and phenylalanine. Its sweetening potential is 180 to 200 times that of saccharose. It has no bitter aftertaste, and several taste tests have attested to its natural flavor. More than sixty countries use it in the production of food and drink products.

Artificial sweeteners have been the topic of many debates over the last few years. Saccharine, especially, has long been considered a carcinogen. However, it does not present the slightest danger if consumed in small daily amounts. (It would only be dangerous after eating 2.5 mg per kilo of body weight, which would correspond to 130 to 160 pounds of sugar for an adult of average weight. Other countries, such as Canada, have outlawed the use of saccharine.

Cyclamates have also been suspected of being carcinogenic, and were outlawed in the United States in 1969. As for aspartame, it has been the object of numerous controversies since its discovery, but every study has proven that it is free of toxins, even when consumed in high doses. The Food and Drug Administration has officially recognized this.

Aspartame is available in two forms:
- in tablets that rapidly dissolve in hot or cold beverages
- in powder form, particularly recommended for desserts and other culinary recipes.

In tablet form, one is as sweet as a 0.2-ounce sugar cube and contains 0.004 ounces of absorbable carbohydrates. In powder form, one teaspoon is as sweet as one teaspoon of sugar and contains 0.14 ounces of absorbable carbohydrates.

In 1980, the accepted daily amount recommended by the World Health Organization was one tablet per pound of body weight. In other words, a person weighing 120 pounds could consume up to 120 tablets in one day without noting any toxic long-term effects. This dose was confirmed in 1984 and in 1987 by the Scientific Committee on Human Diet, the European Economic Community equivalent of the American Food and Drug Administration.

<u>But be careful of artificial sweeteners!</u> Even though we are sure they are non-toxic, they could disturb metabolism in the long run. In effect the body perceives a sweet taste, prepares itself to digest carbohydrates, then cannot find them. If sweeteners are used during the day, any intake of real carbohydrates during those 24 hours could lead to abnormal hyperglycemia, followed by a reactionary hypoglycemia.

Suppose that, "frustrated" by the intake of artificial sweeteners, the body later tries to compensate when carbohydrates are introduced by maximally facilitating their absorption by the intestines. This increased digestive utilization of carbohydrates leads to hyperglycemia (greater than that which normally occurs for the carbohydrate in question) which, by way of the hyperinsulinism set off by it, next leads to hypoglycemia. Thus, hyperinsulinism being a factor in the storage of fats, and hypoglycemia causing a premature return to the sensation of hunger, we are forced to wonder if using artificial sweeteners does not indirectly provoke weight gain. In addition, it must be recognized that the generalization of the use of aspartame in the US over the last 20 years has never been very helpful in preventing the development of obesity in the country.

In fact, we must look at the importance of the taste of sugar. Even if we are certain that it is innate, or at least acquired at a very young age, perhaps while still in the womb, our taste for sugar is often maintained and worsened at even the youngest age. With the help of parents, sweet and sugary become synonymous with love and reward.

It is important to be watchful from the very beginning. Do not excessively promote this love of sugar in your children, and teach them to develop a taste for the sour and bitter tastes. Artificially flavored sodas can serve as a transition from sugary sodas to water for children and adolescents that are "addicted" to sugar. You must persuade yourself that water is the only beverage a child should drink with lunch and dinner. At snack time, fruit juice and skimmed milk are clearly better than soda. In fact, in the end you will want to reverse your child's taste for sugar, and artificial sweeteners may have the opposite effect.

So you must be careful of "dietary delusions." Even as we speak, the food industry is developing proteins that taste like lipids, meant to replace real fats. Faced with these false messages, our bodies may no longer know which tastes to devote themselves to. Because of this, artificial sweeteners should be nothing but transitional because your goal in the long run is to break yourself of your preference for the taste of sugar.

4. Polyols

Polyols, or mass artificial sweeteners, have also appeared in the line of "fake sugars". Their volume complements the recipes of certain products (chocolate, chewing gum and candy) because just a few milligrams of other artificial sweeteners are needed to achieve a sweet taste. Unfortunately, the only advantage polyols have, compared to sugar, is that they do not cause cavities. They have almost the same potential energy as sugar; in the colon, they release fatty acids that are reabsorbed. However, their glycemic index is variable, anywhere from 20 to 65 (the mannitol GI, for instance is one of the lowest). They can even promote, because of fermentation in the colon, bloating and diarrhea.

That means, contrary to what we too often let ourselves believe, their use does not keep us from gaining weight, and they help us even less with losing weight. The "sugar-free" label often hides these polyols: sorbitol, mannitol, xylose, maltose, lactilol, lycasin, polydextrose, etc.

5. Fructose

Compared to polyols, fructose has advantages. The first is that it is not an artificial sweetener with the disadvantages that we have just seen because it can be classified as a "natural sugar". The second is that it has a low glycemic index (20), which goes along well with what we are trying to accomplish. Finally, it has almost the same density as the saccharose in sugar, which makes it easy to use in baking. Just the same, obese people and diabetics must use very moderate amounts because it has been shown that large quantities can raise some people's triglyceride level.

Chapter 10

HOW SHOULD CHILDREN BE FED SO THEY DO NOT GROW UP TO BE OVERWEIGHT?

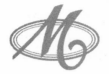

The diet of a small child, especially while he or she is still an infant, should remain the parents' primary concern. During the first month of children's lives, the way in which they eat will condition the state of their health and even their chances of survival.

If problems occur during this time – lack of appetite, vomiting, diarrhea, allergies, etc. – the specialist consulted will not hesitate to analyze the situation, question the baby's diet, and then adjust it. Doctors know perfectly well that in very young children, health problems have always been caused by diet. By adjusting or changing a child's diet, doctors have a much better chance of finding effective solutions by prescribing simple medications.

On the other hand, once children become older, they usually begin to eat "normally", meaning more or less like adults, eating everything or almost everything. At this stage it no longer occurs to parents or doctors that when children are sick, their diets should be reevaluated.

This is unfortunate because most health problems could be resolved by doing so. The appearance of sickness in a child, as with any individual, is first and foremost a sign of physical weakness.

The human body is normally equipped with a natural defense system that protects against germ attacks from its environment. It is said that very young children who put everything in their mouths are "immunized against germs", which really tell us that their system of defense works to protect them from germ invasions.

Yet babies do not have the privilege of having these immune defenses. Children, develop it as they get older (just as for adults), and their bodies use it constantly in order to survive in the surrounding germ-infected environment. Just the same, when the body is weakened, its natural defenses become more vulnerable.

Many sicknesses are the result of a passing weakness in the body which, in most cases, stems from a nutritional problem. That is why children's diets must permanently remain the main concern of parents. Unfortunately the diets of the children of our industrialized countries are rich in quantity, but their quality is becoming worse and worse.

A DEPLORABLE NUTRITIONAL QUALITY

Pondering the ways in which children are fed today, I cannot help but think about the way we feed pets. Some years ago we still made up a "soup" for the dog or cat. Now we just open a can. It is so much more practical. We want to have pets as long as we do not have to take care of them.

That is a yet another illustration of a fundamental characteristic of our era. We want all the advantages without any of the inconvenience. In other words, and according to the famous expression, "We want to have our cake and eat it too."

Most women want to have children. What could be more natural? But in our era, we only want children as long as we do not have to do too much to take care of them. In response to the tendency, we had to organize a sort of industrial breeding system for our charming bambinos, by way of day care centers and professional babysitters. And just as for pets, we had to find practical, industrial solutions for feeding these kids. Now we just have to open a can or box.

Don't worry, I am not so archaic as to refuse all canned food, because some is acceptable. I am rebelling against their common, everyday use. In general, processed food is nutritionally inadequate. So here are the principles I recommend concerning feeding your children. The main objective is to assure their good health, which is a natural consequence of nutritious eating habits.

FOODS TO WATCH

Bread

Just as for adults, children should never eat "white" bread; that is, regular bread made with refined flour. I have already specified that minerals, especially magnesium, are eliminated in the refining process. This process also destroys vitamin B1. We know that this vitamin is indispensable for the metabolism of carbohydrates. A vitamin B deficiency can cause digestive problems and supplementary fatigue. Whole wheat or whole grain bread, contrary to what some say, is not "decalcifying", even when it is unleavened. It even contains a number of minerals and, for children, is usually part of a diet rich in dairy products and, therefore, calcium.

Starches

If your child is of normal build, which would seem to indicate that he or she has a good tolerance for carbohydrates, then there is no reason to deprive him or her of starches. Yet that does not mean that bad carbohydrates, as is too often the case, should become the basis of his or her diet. Systematically resorting to the use of carbohydrates having a high glycemic index, especially potatoes of all kinds and worst of all fries, is usually due to a lack of imagination. In fact it is easy to vary meals without having to spend more money. Reread the tables in Chapter 4, and you will see that there are a number of vegetables that you never even thought of serving.

It is absolutely imperative that you teach your children to eat foods other than bad carbohydrates. Even if they seem to tolerate them at their present age, that will not necessarily be the case when they have finished growing. So it is important to teach them early on to enjoy other foods, especially the other vegetables and legumes we have already talked about.

It is not necessary to give children whole grain pasta. Instead, choose spaghetti and tagliatelle, cooking it just enough so that it maintains, as we saw in previous chapters, a relatively low glycemic index. Avoid pasta made with soft wheat flour (like that found in northern Europe), as well as ravioli or macaroni, which are not extruded.

Also, you do not have to serve them brown rice. It would be better to choose the rice with the lowest glycemic index possible, like Basmati. Get into the habit of always serving rice with vegetables (tomatoes, zucchini, eggplant, peas, cabbage, etc.) as they do in Asia. In India, it is even served with lentils, which is perfect.

Fruit

Children's bodies have resources that adults lost long ago. Therefore they tolerate, without any apparent trouble, food combinations including fruit. So it is possible for children to eat fruit after meals.

On the other hand, as soon as you notice any digestive sensitivity (bloating, stomach aches, or gas) it is best to eliminate fruit during meals. Just as for adults, fruit should be eaten on an empty stomach, especially in the morning when they first wake up, in the evening before going to bed, or as a mid-afternoon snack.

Beverages

Water is, and remains, the only drink that is good for children. Anything that even slightly resembles soft drinks or fruit juice containing corn syrup must absolutely be eliminated because it is a veritable poison for children. In exceptional cases, for a birthday or family party, you can allow your children to drink a few glasses, but firmly remind yourself that it is almost as bad for them as drinking alcohol.

As for cola, we can even say that for children, it is one of the absolute worst for their health because of the level of phosphoric acid, as well as the sugar and caffeine. It could cause serious problems in the strength of your child's bones. Syrups and powdered drink mixes are also discouraged because they contain too much sugar. They accustom children to the taste of sugar, making them dependent upon it. Children can drink fresh fruit juices squeezed at the last minute (so as not to lose the vitamins).

As for milk, it can be drunk during meals, but it is best to choose low-fat milk because of whole milk's bad fat content. In any case, this practice should not continue once the child reaches puberty.

Sugar and sweets

I would not go so far as to totally ban sugar from your children, and yet that would be by far the most reasonable thing to do. I would recommend being very strict when it comes to its consumption.

Besides the sugar they have with breakfast, that which goes on their cereal or in their yogurt, and the sugar in desserts (cookies, pastries, ice cream, etc.), which is already a lot, do not let your children eat sugar in any form. It is necessary to avoid, without necessarily forbidding, all sweets, candy, and chocolate bars, which contain close to 80% sugar. If necessary, reread Chapter 9, dedicated to this subject, in order to convince yourself for good that if sugar is a veritable poison for you, it is that much more so for children.

It is also important to keep young people from becoming dependant upon the taste of sugar. This is important for their immediate health, and indispensable to their future health. I realize that it is difficult to force children to act like regular consumers when they live in an environment that is constantly soliciting them. But that is not a good enough reason to give up, saying there is nothing you can do.

What you can do, at the very least, is establish strict control at home, and above all, teach your children from the very beginning not to become accustomed to the taste of sugar in order to avoid becoming slaves to it. That is why I advise you (contrary to some doctors' opinions) not to give sugar water to infants. It is very easy to accustom them to drinking pure water. When your children are given candy as gifts, treat it as subtly as possible so as to be able to make it completely "disappear" later.

In addition, even if your children's consumption of sweets is modest, it must be completely forbidden before meal. Sugar, in this case, not only ruins their appetite, but also disturbs their glycemia by making it abnormally rise at the beginning of the meal.

Finally, I must remind you one more time that sugar consumption causes vitamin B1 deficiencies. This vitamin, as we have already stressed, is indispensable to the metabolism of carbohydrates. A lack of vitamin B1 forces the body to use its reserves, thus creating a deficit whose consequences are fatigue, difficulty with concentration, attention, and memory, and even a certain form of depression. Thus, it is obvious that your child's schoolwork could seriously suffer.

SHOULD I ALSO REPLACE MY CHILREN'S SUGAR WITH ARTIFICIAL SWEETENERS?

If adults are advised to replace sugar with artificial sweeteners from time to time (with the caution we raised in the previous chapter), why not do so for children? This is a good question.

If the child is truly overweight for his or her age, you may resort to artificial sweeteners only in a transition period. If, on the other hand, the child's build is normal, there is no reason to categorically eliminate the couple of teaspoons he or she uses at breakfast of in yogurt.[20]

In order to limit your daily sugar intake (and this recommendation refers to the whole family), you can prepare desserts with artificial sweeteners or fructose. That said, let us look now at how you can organize your children's meals.

---

[20] You can also replace white sugar (saccharose) with fructose, which can be found in stores and whose glycemic index is much lower.

MEALS

The objectives we must reach for in making up children's menus are the following:

Avoid overloading the menu bad carbohydrates in order to keep the body from secreting abnormal amounts of insulin. That could cause future hyperinsulinism, the open door to weight gain, diabetes, and cardiovascular disease.

On the subject of diet, everyone will tell you with great conviction – because it usually shows good sense – that you must serve "balanced meals." That usually means meals that contain proteins, carbohydrates and lipids.

Of course. But it is important to know what goes under each of these headings.

It is true. You must eat proteins, carbohydrates, lipids and fiber to be sure to absorb all the substances your body needs. This is particularly true for growing children. On the other hand, the error that most of us make – even in the medical world – is believing that the meal itself will bring us this dietary balance. When we speak of balanced meals, we should mention that this balance should be attained throughout the entire day, that is, over the course of several meals instead of just one. That makes all the difference.

BREAKFAST

Anglo-Saxons are correct in considering breakfast the most important meal of the day. This is particularly true for children. But we have yet to determine how it should ideally be composed. My recommendation is to make your children's breakfast a meal in which *good carbohydrates* are the main focus.

You could serve, in no specific order:

- Bread, preferably whole wheat, on which you could spread a little butter. Ban the regular peanut butter which is full of sugar and bad carbohydrates. Instead, use a sugar free one.
- Cereal (multi-grain if possible; avoid corn flakes and any other cereal containing corn, sugar, honey or caramel)
- Fresh fruit
- Reduced sugar or, even better, sugar-free preserves
- Dairy products (milk, yogurt)

I discourage honey for children who are bordering on overweight because the concentration of high-glycemic index sugar (even though it is natural for honey) is much too great. Others can use moderate amounts of honey.

LUNCH

Lunch will focus on proteins. Inevitably, it will thus contain meat or fish. The ideal would be to avoid systematically serving carbohydrates with a high glycemic index with meat and fish as we normally do. It is best to avoid French fries, baked potatoes (index 95) and even mashed potatoes (index 90). Potatoes boiled in their skins are completely acceptable as well as sweet potatoes.

The other vegetables should also be chosen from among those whose glycemic index is low (beans, lentils, peas, chickpeas, sweet potatoes, etc.) or even moderate (Basmati rice or semolina). Taking into account their low carbohydrate concentration, there is no reason why cooked carrots should be restricted from children.

Still, get into the habit of serving, in addition to everything else, fiber-rich vegetables (beans, cauliflower, mushrooms, etc.). Do not always give your children the same thing to eat. It is important for them to become accustomed to eating a varied diet. Unfortunately, school age children may eat lunch away from home and very probably at the school cafeteria. In that case, you will not have control over what your children eat. However, if they are not "too fat", the situation will not be that dramatic. You just have to adjust their dinner.

SNACKS

For all people in general and children in particular, it is best to increase the number of meals rather than decrease it. Just like for breakfast, snacks will mostly contain carbohydrates. If you give your children bread, it is best to serve it whole wheat or made with unrefined flour. You can put a little butter on it if you wish or sugar free peanut butter. Finally, you could give your child a chocolate bar, but only one of good quality, containing at least 70% cacao.

DINNER

Your child's dinner should be, as it was for lunch, based on meat, fish, eggs, or even "good" carbohydrates such as lentils, Basmati rice or pasta. Yet no matter what option you choose, the first course of the child's meal should be a thick vegetable soup, made of leeks, tomatoes, celery, etc.

Children generally do not eat enough green vegetables because they do not like the taste since they have not been trained appropriately. Yet they contain fiber, which is indispensable to good bowel functioning, as well as vitamins, minerals, and trace elements. The best way to get them to eat vegetables is to have them eat them in a good vegetable soup.

There is yet a third category of meals that is perfect for children and that they love: stuffed vegetables, such as tomatoes, eggplant, zucchini, artichokes, or cabbage. In effect, this is a very simple way to incorporate fiber-rich vegetables, allowing you to broaden your choices from the eternal pizza, pasta, rice, and potatoes.

With dinner, serve light dairy products made with low-fat milk for dessert, such as custard or crème caramel, lightly sweetened or made with fructose. You could also end the meal with plain yogurt flavored with a little sugar-free jam. Every once in a while they can eat a classic piece of cake on special occasions.

I recommend that you completely exclude one kind of food from your house: hamburgers and hotdogs. You will not be able to keep your child from liking hamburgers any more than soft drinks, but this is not a good enough reason to make them for him or her at home. This type of food is bad for your health because it contains too many bad carbohydrates and an excess of dangerous saturated fats.

Reserve this type of food for occasions that call for practical ways to fee your family, which is often the case when you are away from home. Hamburgers and hotdogs originally were invented in America because they were quickly prepared and eaten either at work when people could not leave for lunch or dinner, or on trips, which are always long in an immense country like the United States. Eating a hamburger or hotdog at home is as ridiculous as sleeping on a cot in a sleeping bag, and it also puts your health at risk.

So avoid falling into this deplorable extreme for the sake of convenience, which is unfortunately already the case for most people in a large number of countries, some of them among the most civilized, where some children do not even know what a normal meal is. Only take your children to the sadly famous fast food restaurants on very exceptional occasions if they like them or to not waste time if you are on a trip, but this should not become a habit. To reward your children, would it not be more reasonable to take them to a good restaurant to give them a taste for "la grande cuisine", especially French?

On the other hand, it is quite possible to make things at home that will remind your children of "fast food." For example you can make a pizza by making the crust yourself from whole grain flour, like buckwheat. As far as pizza is concerned, never buy this thick crust pizza. Choose only pizza with the thinnest crust. You could also make crepes from the same type of flour. If, for practical reasons, you must make sandwiches, avoid peanut butter-and-jelly on white bread. Instead, choose whole wheat bread and ham (as lean as possible), cheese, fish (smoked salmon), and a little lettuce or tomato.

SPECIAL CASES

Overweight children

Some children are charged with a few extra pounds very early on, but not so much so that their parents worry about it enough to take them to a doctor. Still, if they decide to do so, most doctors will say that those few extra pounds do not make the child obese. In addition, they will stress, and rightfully so, that no low-calorie diet is even imaginable for a growing child. Nine times out of ten, doctors will reassure the parents, saying that when the child gets taller, especially at the start of adolescence, he or she will be of normal weight for their age.

Just the same, know that excess weight in children is, in all cases, an obvious sign of problems with metabolism. Take it seriously if your child is overweight because if the problem is addressed in time, it will be quite easy to reestablish a healthy balance. For children, as for adults, excessive stored fats indicate poor glucose tolerance. The dietary principles outlined in the Method (Chapter 4) should be applied. That will essentially mean eliminating all carbohydrates whose glycemic index is greater than 50. If the child eats a bad carbohydrate at some point, it is best to automatically compensate for the potential elevation in glycemia by adding a carbohydrate whose glycemic index is very low.

Once the child has reached a normal weight it will be possible, as it is for adults, to progressively reintegrate a few bad carbohydrates with a high glycemic index, meaning exceptions that you will have to manage. It is true that with puberty, some overweight boys get progressively thinner without necessarily changing their diet. At this point in their lives, adolescents use huge amounts of energy, and they generally engage in intense physical activity.

Exercise must be encouraged because it can prevent the onset of obesity or help to reduce it. It has been show that for children, excess weight is proportional to the number of hours spent in front of the television during the day (encouraging inactivity, snacking, and ads for products that are not very nutritious). Be careful because teenage boys who were overweight when they were younger are invariably candidates for being overweight once they have finished growing.

For girls, the situation is generally the opposite. The risk of weight gain appears during puberty, when their bodies are becoming more woman-like. The female body is very sensitive, and any variation of the hormonal system (during puberty, pregnancy and menopause) is a risk factor in the balance of metabolism. Young girls and women are perfectly aware of this but, worried about maintaining their "figure", unfortunately adopt diets that cause them to starve, invariably leading to depression or anorexia and bulimia. Young girls whose weight puberty tends to affect can, without any worry whatsoever, adopt the dietary principles of this book. Not only can they maintain their "figure", but they will also gain a sense of vitality, perfect for their desire to "conquer the world".

Tired children

Are you not shocked by how today's children and adolescents are more and more tired and lethargic, painfully dragging themselves from the bed to the couch? Remember that an excess of bad carbohydrates at breakfast will set of hypoglycemia around 11 o'clock with sleepiness, lack of concentration, yawning, apathy or aggressiveness, signs that teachers frequently notice in their classrooms near the end of the morning.

This phenomenon could repeat itself throughout the day if, at lunch, the child abuses French fries, white bread and soft drinks. Sugary snacks containing fats, like cakes and pastries, will even further affect this.

Next the child, back at home, often installs him or herself in front of the television which, (a number of studies have shown it) encourages snacking and incites these young, impressionable minds to consume sweets or cookies. The park would certainly be more beneficial for them than this "living room sport". A diet that is not diverse enough often causes children to detest fiber-rich foods (fruits, vegetables and legumes), even though the foods that contain them are rich in vitamins, minerals and trace elements. All of these shortages are factors leading to asthenia (weakness or loss of strength).

Chapter 11

DIET AND EXERCISE

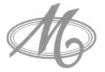

If you should walk around the streets of New York, Los Angeles, or any other city in America before daybreak, you would not be able to help noticing the people sweating blood and water, already at 5:00 a.m. Despite the extreme pollution of which their activated lungs cheerfully take advantage before the sun is even up, these sportsmen and women sacrifice themselves to their ritual, perfect examples of the American citizen.

Except for a few pseudo-marathoners, the large majority of these morning maniacs think that vigorous daily exercise is enough to guarantee them tip-top shape and keep them from looking like the Michelin Man. America has been trying to get in shape for years, and despite the rise in its citizens' average weight, they remain convinced that the best way to lose weight is to take in fewer and burn more calories.

Much more reasonably, Parisians are happy to walk around the lake in the Bois de Boulogne a few times every Saturday morning.

This also gives them their weekly oxygen fix, even if it is just enough to regain their strength, (which they had not necessarily lost, by the way). In 1989, a poll taken by a large French weekly indicated that 66% of French people think that the best way to lose weight is through exercise.

This is a preconceived idea that is even more surprising in that those who have tried it have rarely succeeded. It is purely illusory to try to lose weight without changing your eating habits.

We cannot deny that exercise increases energy expenditure, but that expenditure is, in fact, much smaller than we think.

CONTINUOUS EXERCISE	TIME IT TAKES TO LOSE 2 LBS. OF FAT BY EXERCISING	
	MEN (hours)	WOMEN (hours)
Walking at a normal pace	138	242
Walking rapidly	63	96
Golf	36	47
Bicycling	30	38
Swimming (crawl)	17	21
Jogging	14	18
Tennis	13	16
Squash	8	11

Source: Dr. Mondenard

Studies done by a certain Dr. Mondenard show that losing 2 pounds through exercise would take several hours. So, a person wanting to lose 11 pounds just through exercise would have to jog for an hour and a half nonstop, five times a week.

Endurance pays!

What all exercise candidates should know is that it is the prolonged effort beyond a certain point that permits you to obtain results in weight loss. That is why one hour of continuous muscle work will be much more effective than thirty minutes three times a day. While at rest, the body uses fatty acids in the blood as well as the muscles' ATP (adenosine triphosphate) for fuel.

As soon as intense physical exercise begins, the body delves into muscular glycogen for fuel, which would run out in around twenty minutes if that were all the body was counting on. After the first 25 minutes of exercise, half of the energy used will become glycogen, and the other half will be used in the transformation of stored fats (lipolysis). After forty minutes of work, mostly fats are used, so as to protect the remaining glycogen. So it is only after that first forty minutes of continuous effort at almost maximum intensity that you begin to "burn" stored fat.

You now understand that if you do twenty minutes of exercise three times daily, the glycogen your body uses for fuel has time to build itself back up by drawing its energy directly from food, and you do not burn stored fat. To obtain real results, you must do an endurance exercise (biking, jogging or swimming) at least three times a week, maintaining the activity level for at least forty minutes. A three-day interruption will cancel all the previously obtained efforts.

Moreover, it is important for those who exercise to adopt a diet that conforms to the principles of this book, notably in order to eliminate all risk of hypoglycemia.[21] It is equally necessary to begin slowly, not prolonging the duration of the exercise all at once without training. The body needs time to get used to the physiological change gradually.

---

[21] The athlete's diet is much more complex and calls for other nutritional rules that are specific to each type of sport, too specific to be addressed in this book.

Exercise can be beneficial

In effect, it can be beneficial if intelligently practiced, with the principal end goal being good health and better oxygenation. In fact, it could almost be said that the human body (like all of its functions) "only wears out if we do not use it." Physical exercise is a form of permanent regeneration that helps the body to, among other things, fight against aging by improving cardiac and pulmonary functioning. Even if your weight remains the same, you will have a slimmer figure because little by little, muscle will replace fat.

Muscular activity can also be an effective aid in the "restoration" of our bodies, meaning that same "getting into shape" that we have undertaken by following the recommendations of this book. It is important to know that glucose tolerance improves and hyperinsulinism (cause of hypoglycemia and obesity) is significantly diminished. It is especially along these lines that exercise is useful, accelerating the correction of hyperinsulinism. We can add that arterial hypertension and hypercholesterolemia are clearly improved.

On a psychological level, reasonable amounts of exercise can be quite beneficial. You will rediscover your body and gain a sense of youthfulness. Exercise rapidly becomes, with the improvement of your performance, a veritable source of well being. By generally improving your metabolism, physical activity can not only help you to lose weight, but also guarantee weight stabilization and health maintenance.

Do not lose sight of the objective.

Unfortunately, our attitudes are sometimes too extreme when it comes to exercise. Between the pseudo-athletic smoker/boozer who spends the third half of the game at the bar or in front of the television, and the old beau who is dying to stay young, exercising as if he were a professional athlete, there is only one good way to exercise that only wisdom will lead you to discover.

Monday morning work absences are not only due to weekend alcohol abuse and other dietary excesses. They can also be attributed to the carelessness of many who, not used to or trained in a sport and not drinking enough water, have misjudged, in their euphoria, their true capabilities. A combination of healthy diet management and reasonable, regular physical activity is what you need in order to accept your accumulating years with serenity, youth, and optimism.

When you see people who insist on waiting five minutes for the elevator just to go to the second floor, or taking their car to go buy cigarettes at the next-door market, you can only feel the same sense of pity for them as you do for people who only eat hamburgers and drink cola.

Chapter 12

IDEAL WEIGHT

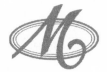

When we weigh ourselves, what are we measuring? The answer is the total weight of our bones, muscles, fat, organs, viscera, nerves and water. Fat makes up about 15% of men's weight, and about 22% of women's. Obesity is defined as an excess of this body fat, surpassing average weight by at least 20%. But how can we measure the exact amount of fat in the body? Measuring the thickness of a fold of skin with a compass is one approach among many, but it is not very precise.

We normally associate obesity with excess weight, even if the scale does not differentiate between fatty mass and active mass (muscles, organs, etc.). Instead of referring to weight charts severely established by insurance companies, it is much simpler to figure out your ideal weight using the Lorentz formula (height in cm and weight in kg):

$$\text{Weight (men)} = (\text{Height} - 100) - \frac{(\text{Height} - 150)}{4}$$

$$\text{Weight (women)} = (\text{Height} - 100) - \frac{(\text{Height} - 140)}{2}$$

But this calculation does not take into account either age or skeletal structure, and it is not valid for petite women (shorter than 1.50 m or about 5 ft.). It is best to resort to the weight at which you feel best, which everyone senses intuitively. The Quetelet index or BMI (Body Mass Index) is often used nowadays. It is the relationship between weight and height squared.

$$\text{Index} = \frac{\text{Weight (in kg)}}{\text{Height}^2 \text{ (in m}^2)}$$

The average BMI for men is between 20 and 25. For women it is between 19 and 24. From the upper limits to 29, one is slightly overweight. From 30 on, one is obese, and if the index is greater than 40, one is seriously obese and has a serious medical problem. The BMI is medical, not aesthetic, but it has the advantage of being fairly accurate in the calculation of fatty mass.

Today, special scales exist that not only calculate weight but also body fat. They are useful for following your progressive loss of fatty mass. Because becoming thin means losing weight, but especially melting away stored fats.

The topographical distribution of fats permits us to evaluate the seriousness of obesity. This distribution is measured using the following formula:

$$\frac{\text{Waist measurement (at the navel)}}{\text{Hip measurement (at fullest part)}}$$

We can simple calculate the index with the help of the following table:

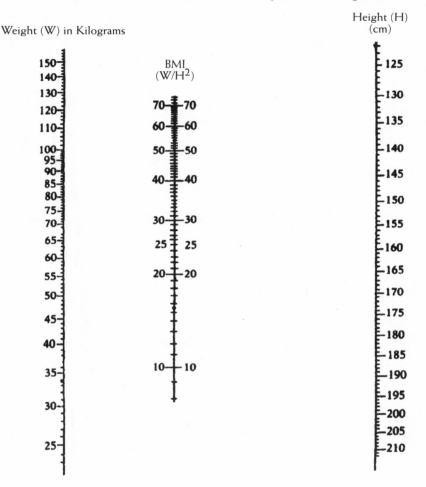

The index is found on the line between weight and height.

It is generally 0.85-1 for men and 0.65-0.85 for women. In androgenic obesity, most fat is concentrated in the upper body (face, neck and abdomen below the waist). The ratio is always greater than one. Its complications show up early and are frequent: diabetes, hypercholesterolemia, high blood pressure and cardiovascular diseases.

In gynecoid obesity, most of the fatty mass is found in the lower body (hips, buttocks, thighs and lower belly). This distribution is normally found in the female body. The risk of illness is less. The problem is more aesthetic. Cellulite is often present in this type of obesity.

Beyond the medical statistics, which try to scientifically quantify what is more an aesthetic concern or discomfort, the most important weight for the patient to concentrate on is the one he or she wishes to achieve, the one that feels the most comfortable. In sum, the goal should be the weight that provides the patient with a sense of well-being.

This weight is sometimes above theoretical norms, but why be stricter than the obese person is? If this number seems to him or her to be possible to achieve, it is more realistic than the theoretical norm imposed by the medical world which, if too strict, can be a form of discouragement from the very start. On the other hand, women must be aware of images that are often overly influenced by the media. These images cause women to set mythical, unrealistic goals that are impossible to attain. Women's bodies are fully equipped with reasonable regulatory systems that will prevent them from reaching such a point. The ideal weight, if such a thing exists, must be carefully thought out, sometimes with the critical help of a doctor.

CONCLUSION

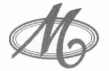

As we know, humans have existed on earth for more than three million years.

The homo erectus, then homo sapiens were essentially hunters, fishermen, and gatherers. The dietary portion of primitive humans was thus composed of a significant amount of fat proteins, but also of carbohydrates in the form of berries in the spring and summer, and roots in the fall and winter.

Human waste found by archeologists shows very sinewy excrement, due to a significant fiber concentration. This indicates, then, that primitive and prehistoric humans' diets had a very low glycemic index.

During the mesolithic period (10,000 BC), humans began to domesticate certain wild grains. In several milleniums, they settled and devoted themselves to agriculture.

That is why in Egypt wheat and lentils were cultivated. More to the north, the Celts and Saxons cultivated oats and millet, but also rye and buckwheat.

All of these grains and legumes are consumed in their original state, without undergoing refinement. All induce low glycemias.

And it is in this way that during the 10 to 12 millenniums that preceded us, the human diet was enriched with new species during their domestication, but also with migratory population influxes, the development of large civilizations, and their immense brewing.

But in the end, even if humans had a more diversified diet, its nature had not changed since the mists of time since its carbohydrate contribution was barely glycemic.

Yet since the beginning of the 19th century, and for the first time in the entire history of humanity, humans began to introduce on a large scale into the ancestral dietary style of their contemporaries, new or transformed foods that had perverse metabolic effects.

If all of a sudden on January 1, 1820, an experiment had been done in a western country, by giving to a representative sample of the population of the time, to be consumed during an entire year: sugar, potatoes, and white flour, in the proportions we consume with impunity today (50 to 100 times more for sugar), or under the hyperglycemiant forms in which we still eat them (hyper-refined flour, fries and au gratin potatoes), the undesirable side effects on the public health by the end of the year would have been evident to everyone, and everybody would have seen the relationship between cause and effect. Without a single doubt, the authorities would have taken the measures necessary for prohibiting the production and consumption of these products, by invoking the obvious reasons of public health.

But as the introduction of these perverse products occured quite progressively in the different levels of the population, the metabolic effects induced only began to appear quite a long time later.

How could one, in effect, more than a century later, when in 1930 one began to pay attention to the quite relative obesity in the United States, imagine the slow, insidious process that had been initiated at the beginning of the previous century?

If Thérèse Desqueyroud, the famous character of Nobel laureate novelest François Mauriac, had given her husband a large glass of cyanide as soon as she had decided to get rid of him, he would have been dead on the spot. The poisoning thesis would have been immediately verified, and guilty Thérèse would have been unmasked. But by giving him the poison in small doses over long months, the criminal simply made her husband a sick person whose symptoms did not reveal their true cause to the doctors of the time. Thus the crime was perfect, since no cause-effect relationship could be established.

It is somewhat this same type of scenario, though obviously on a different scale, that has occured with obesity. But it is particularly dramatic to discover today that it is precisely a very short amount of time after having identified the symptoms of a serious illness (obesity) a half a century ago that the factors responsible for its true cause (hyperinsulinism) were paradoxically reinforced and developed.

In June 1944, the Americans debark on the coasts of Normandy to liberate France from German occupation. In their bags they have tons of provisions, made and loaded months earlier. To assure that these products would be well-preserved, certain procedures (industrial treatments, conditioning) were invented to better respond to the demands of the circumstances.

Flour was hyper-refined to assure better shelf-life, and potatoes were dehydrated and reduced into flakes to take up less space, something which had never been done before.

But what we did not know was that all operations initiated for obvious practical reasons had the effect of considerably increasing the glycemic index of the main ingredient. And just as the Parmentier's potato had been in the beginning "a temporary substitute" to the lack of wheat, these new products, instead of being placed in the post-war surplus stores, were not only conserved but generalized. They were even becoming the precursors of an interminable generation of refined and industrialized products that would completely transform the dietary prospect of the second half of the 20th century. And what no one knew and could not even imagine is that these products, like their regrettable hyperglycemic predecessors, were going to make worse a situation of metabolic perturbation that was already close to the danger mark.

With hindsight, we thus realize that for close to two centuries the human race was progressively adopting, without knowing, a dietary mode that was incompatible with the genetic heritage of its metabolism.

Once again, for more than three million years, the pancreases of humans, at first primitive, then prehistoric, then those of the Middle Ages, the Renaissance and even the Industrial Revolution, were barely used. In addition, it was not necessary for this organ to be capable of supporting excessive stimulations because hyperglycemic food did not exist.

The pancreas with which humans are genetically equipped today is thus the result of a history of use (old by several hundreds of millenniums) which is somehow our metabolic heritage. Just as it is impossible for a human to look at the sun directly because his or her eyes are not able to endure it, it is impossible to impunitively stimulate the insulinic function of our pancreas beyond its natural physiological limits.

Weight gain leading to being overweight, even to obesity, is thus simply the consequence of the abusive stimulation of a key metabolic organ because of an inappropriate dietary mode for which the human body was not genetically programmed.

We thus understand now that it is the effect induced by a slow and insidious derivative of our western dietary habits since the beginning of the 19th century, and especially these last fifty years, that is at the origin of the endemic obesity of our era.

As long as this realization has not been made and the suitable recommendations have not been formulated in an official way, hyperinsulinism will remain one of the dominating pathologies of our modern era with, as a consequence, not only a generalization of obesity, but also of diabetes and cardio-vascular illnesses.

The modest pretention of this work is thus to permit the reader to discover that it is sufficient to learn to eat better by making appropriate dietary choices, not only to become and remain thin, but also and especially to rediscover a satisfying level of health and maintain it for always.

Appendix I

CRITICISMS OF
THE MONTIGNAC METHOD

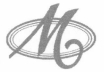

A certain number of criticisms of the Montignac Method have been voiced here and there. They especially come from people (nutritionists, dieticians and journalists) who have a poor overall understanding of the Method, never having taken the time to seriously dwell on the subject (most never even read the book). Others have deliberately presented an oversimplified, caricatured picture of the author so as to discredit him, and many only refer to the first edition of the book (1987), refusing to recognize the continual evolution of the Montignac Method demonstrated in the six successive editions of the book.

So here is a good place for me to address the principal allegations made against the Method.

Is the Montignac Method a dissociation diet?

Some tendentious presentations, in effect, call the Montignac Method a dissociation diet. As Professor Apfelbaum explains in his article called "Diététique et Nutrition", a dissociation diet consists of only eating one type of food per day. You would eat chicken for all three meals on Monday, pasta on Tuesday, cheese on Wednesday, vegetables on Thursday, fish on Friday, etc.

For those of you who have just finished reading "Eat Yourself Slim," it is more than evident that the Montignac Method has nothing to do with the dissociation gimmick.

Is the Montignac Method inspired by the Hay Method?

The Montignac Method's vocation is to provide a way for those who have a weight problem to lose a substantial amount of weight for good, and to get into better physical and intellectual shape. The scientific bases for the Method correspond to discoveries made during the 1970s and 80s on the <u>metabolism of carbohydrates and lipids. The physio-pathology of its principles is based on the very precise notions of hyperinsulinism, hyperglycemia, and the classification of carbohydrates based on their carbohydrate concentration</u>.

The Hay Method, on the other hand, is based on beliefs that date back to the end of the nineteenth century. Following it means avoiding certain combinations of food, for example, carbohydrates and proteins, to prevent intoxicating the blood. The objective of the Hay Method (whose principles are completely invalidated by modern scientific knowledge) is mostly to cure, or at least prevent, certain diseases of the arteries and digestive problems.

It is total fantasy to say that the Montignac Method is a replica of the Hay Method, even though Hay, who was rather sensible, also advised eating fruit on an empty stomach for those who had digestive problems.

Is the Montignac Method inspired by the Atkins diet?

The Atkins diet was all the rage in the 60s and 70s after its founder said that all foods were good except carbohydrates. At the time, he suspected insulin of being the "catalyst" of weight gain. But since he thought that all carbohydrates induced the same glycemia, Dr. Atkins recommended definitively excluding them from our diets.

This diet of exclusion led those who followed it to consume too much fat because he made no restrictions on it. In addition, at that time we did not yet know the difference between good fats and bad fats. As a result, there was a surge of cardiovascular problems in people who had followed the Atkins diet, which came to be known as a "passport to heart attacks".

Calling the Montignac Method a "watered-down Atkins diet", as do some misleading commentators, is intentionally deceiving. In fact, the Montignac Method recommends consuming a number of carbohydrates, as long as their glycemic index is low: fruit, vegetables, whole grains, and spaghetti. In addition, the kind of fat to be consumed is clearly specified to assure effective prevention (see Chapter 8).

Is there cardiovascular risk in the Montignac Method?

The popular success of the Montignac Method is sometimes seen as a threat to certain professions. In effect, it can bring up questions of the credibility of professional nutritionists who continue to refer to inexact, ineffective, and outdated notions like the caloric ration or the erroneous classification of carbohydrates into slow sugars and fast sugars.

An official poll published in Holland by the GFK Institute has shown that because of the influence of the Montignac Method's nutritional messages, the country's consumption of sugar decreased by 25% and of potatoes by 14% in 1997. Let us also note that the study specified that the consumption of whole grains, green vegetables and fruit had considerably risen because of the Montignac Method's nutritional influence. "Thanks to Montignac," said another study, the Dutch drink less beer and more red wine.

Statistical information like this can cause certain professions to worry. That is why it is completely understandable that as soon as the development of the Montignac Method is somehow felt as a threat to the interests of the members of a corporation, certain negative rumors are intentionally started and publicly spread. This was what happened in countries where the notoriety of the Method became a veritable national affair.

But in most cases, the criticisms of the Method came from people who wanted to deliberately harm the notoriety of the author. In addition, on different occasions we were able to catch these people blatantly lying, or at least show that they had, for the most part, a complete misunderstanding of the Method.

In 1996, a nutritionist was invited to represent those "against Montignac" on the popular Belgian television show, "La Balle au Centre". She found herself forced to publicly admit that she had never read a book by Montignac but that in her reviews she just reported the opinions of her colleagues, whom she said knew the Montignac Method well.

Since they cannot deny the efficacy of the said Method because it is obvious that the resulting weight loss is substantial and long lasting, its opponents have concentrated their criticisms around their so-called cardiovascular risks. They also claim (as does Dr. Jacques Fricker, main opponent among the French) that the Montignac Method being "too fatty" (because it eliminates, according to them, carbohydrates), it raises cardiovascular risk in general, and cholesterol in particular.

To say that the Montignac Method is "too fatty" is obviously totally false because two independent studies have shown the opposite to be true:
- In 1994, the Center for the Study and Information of Vitamins, in France showed that patients who follow the Montignac Method consumed 31.2% lipids.
- The work of Canadian Professors Dumesnil and Tremlay (see p. 227) showed a 32% fat intake.
- "Classical" nutritionists recommend a 30% fat intake, and the average French person consumes 40 to 42% fats. Again, total fat content is less important than the types of fats you choose.

In early 1998, young Dutch doctors of Eindhoven Hospital went so far as to uphold the rumor that some patients following the Montignac Method had experienced small heart attacks. This grave information (never verified or confirmed, of course) was spread by unscrupulous and sensationalist journalists, to the point where they even made people believe there had been deaths. A few weeks later, the rumor having traversed the frontiers, a large Catalonian newspaper in Barcelona clearly implied that, "several people had died of heart attacks in Holland after having (according to certain rumors) followed the Montignac Method; the Dutch Minister of Health had (according to other rumors) 'prohibited the practice.'"

Even though this type of news is both deceitful and slanderous, it is just the same enough to destabilize some of those who had faith in the Method and to discourage the rest. As Beaumarchais said in **The Barber of Seville**, "Slander, slander, there will always be something left."

Even though we must treat this gossip with contempt, it is useful to respond to it, if only to further stress the vile intentions of its creators. Regularly, journalists who do their job honestly ask their questions this way, "Is it possible that following the Montignac Method could lead to an increase in cardiovascular risk, in particular a rise in cholesterol?"

Our response is the following:

First, let us note that all of Michel Montignac's books are prefaced by renowned professors and cardiovascular specialists:

- Professor Maurice Cloarec, Head of Cardiology at the Hôpital Tenon in Paris, who noticed in his consultations a very clear decline in the cholesterol of those who followed the recommendations of the first book, *Comment maigrir en faisant des repas d'affaires* (the original French version of *Dine Out and Lose Weight*).

- Dr. Morrison Bethea, cardiovascular surgeon who reports that his patients ended up lowering their cholesterol by 30 to 40%.

- Professor Jean Dumesnil, from the Institut de Cardiologie of the Hôpital Laval in Quebec, who claimed that in a 1997 experiment, following the Montignac Method was shown to be a powerful factor in preventing cardiovascular risk.

- Dr. Hervé Robert, Professor at the Paris University and Director at the Institut Vitalité et Nutrition in Paris, is gathering claims made by hundreds of doctors who proscribe the Montignac Method every day in their offices. His colleagues consistently note at the same time weight loss, an improvement in total cholesterol level, LDL cholesterol, HDL cholesterol, triglycerides, glycemia, insulin, etc.

What is more, among the thousands of testimonies received from readers over the last ten years, not one of them ever mentioned a rise in cholesterol as a result of following the Montignac Method. On the contrary, most people with high cholesterol reported a substantial reduction.

In addition, all nutritionists know, because it was demonstrated a long time ago, that all forms of weight loss (no matter what the Method) automatically lead to a drop in cholesterol. You must then be of bad faith (especially if you are a doctor) to claim that the Montignac Method increases the risk of hypercholesterolemia, even though we also recognize that it leads to an undeniable loss of weight.

Moreover, commentators on the Montignac Method (whether for or against it) are unanimous in recognizing that one of the Method's greatest merits is that it rehabilitates a diet rich in fiber, especially soluble fiber. All the studies on cholesterol have shown that it slowly decreases with the introduction of fiber into the diet. There again, you must be of bad faith to say that, "Montignac makes your cholesterol go up," even though we recognize that his diet is quite rich in fiber.

In Michel Montignac's books, it has never been said, like some deceitfully claim without having read the books, that you had to eat <u>more</u> fat. All the books, in fact, contain an important chapter on preventing cardiovascular risk where very precise food choices are recommended, especially:
- to eat as few saturated fats as possible
- to choose mono unsaturated fats (olive oil, goose and duck fat) and polyunsaturated fats, especially those in the omega 3 family (fish fats).

According to the American "Nurses' Health Study," the prevention of coronary diseases <u>is more effective</u> if one replaces dietary fats with other fats than if one reduces total fat intake. It is thus not the amount of fat that matters, but its <u>quality</u>. Professor Stampfer confirmed this when he showed that even thought 45% of the calories consumed by the inhabitants of Crete come from fats, the fact that these fats come almost exclusively from olive oil explains why the rate of cardiovascular illness in this country is the lowest in the world.

It has also been shown that two of the major risk factors for cardiovascular illness, especially hypertension, were hyperinslinism and insulin resistance. A number of researchers, among them Jenkins, have shown that by reducing insulinemia, we reduce cardiovascular risk. Moreover, J.C. Brand Miler has shown that a diet containing low glycemic indexes lowers cholesterol by 6% and triglycerides by 9%. In the same way, this researcher showed that sugar consumption lead to a rise in bad cholesterol (LDL cholesterol) and a drop in good cholesterol (HDL cholesterol).

Everyone knows that the basic principle of the Montignac Method consists of, besides eliminating sugar (among other bad carbohydrates), opting for foods having a low glycemic index (legumes, fruit, whole grains, spaghetti, etc.) consequentially lowering insulinemia.

Also, as far as lipids are concerned, fatty acids are chosen with precision to assure optimal cardiovascular prevention. Here again, it is not easy to see how the application of the principles of the Montignac Method could have inverse results (increased cardiovascular risk) since all studies have shown that the application of such principles precisely resulted in a significant drop in risk.

Consequently, wanting to attribute any rise in cardiovascular risk to following the Montignac Method reveals specific intentions. Taking into account the hundreds of thousands of individuals who may feel led to follow the Montignac Method, no matter what country they come from, we cannot deny the fact that a person who has already had cardiovascular problems can have a heart attack, despite following the Montignac Method. But the claim, without obvious proof, of a cause-and-effect relationship between the two, like the one made by a Dutch practitioner, says much about the critic's desire to discredit any notoriety (that of Montignac) that might disrupt his or her corporation.

Appendix II

SPECIAL ADVICE TO VEGETARIANS

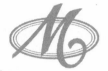

If love and respect for animals are what motivate vegetarians to not eat meat, it is completely respectable. If, on the other hand, the argument is based on the idea that meat is a source of hazardous "toxins," then it is reasoning founded on notions of physiology dating back to the nineteenth century that are outdated today.

These famous toxins do not add up to much because they simply refer to the uric acid and urea that develop in the body after protein consumption, whether the protein came from meat or not. It is important to know that these substances are completely eliminated by the kidneys of normal subjects who drink enough fluids. The body, which in reality is "programmed" to eliminate these metabolic waste products, does its job rather well, and without damage. The eventual "clogging" of which some people speak is therefore unfounded.

Vegetarians, who do not eat meat, sausage, poultry, or fish, must still maintain a sufficient intake of animal by-products in order to balance their diet correctly. To do this, they will have to opt for dairy products and eggs. To properly cover these protein needs, you must have a good knowledge of nutrition and know, for example, that animal proteins and vegetable proteins are not identical and that some are only partially assimilated by the body.

Vegetable proteins do not have the same nutritional value as animal proteins, and 10g of protein from lentils will not have the same value as 10g of egg protein. These notions are indispensable for those who wish to maintain proper protein intake, keeping in mind that one should have 1g of protein per day per 2 lb. of body weight.

Those vegetarians who are also "grand amateurs" of soy should know that not all soy foods contain the same amount of protein. Proteins contained in different soy foods, for 3.5 oz.:
- Soy flour: 45g
- Soy grain: 35g
- Tofu: 13g
- Soy germ: 4g
- Soy sprouts: 1.5g

You should also know that soy juice, mistakenly called "soy milk" is rather low in calcium (42 mg per 4 ounces) compared to cow's milk (120 mg per 4 ounces). In addition, vegetable proteins are lower in essential amino acids (those that the body does not produce on its own), grains are low in lysine and legumes in methionine. On this last point, you will learn that it is important to combine whole grains, legumes and oleaginous fruits (walnuts, hazelnuts, almonds, etc.) on a daily basis.

Moreover, a number of ancient exotic dishes systematically mix grains and legumes:
- corn and kidney beans in Mexican tortillas,

- semolina and chickpeas in Maghrebian couscous,
- meal and peanuts in black Africa.

On the other hand eggs alone contain a very rich and perfect balance of amino acids.

Vegetarians must pay special attention to their iron intake, keeping in mind that vegetable iron is five times harder for the body to assimilate than animal iron. In order to avoid vitamin B12 deficiencies, you will have to be sure to include cheese, eggs and seaweed in your diet.

Well-planned vegetarian meals are totally acceptable and can even be particularly beneficial in the prevention of cardiovascular risk and certain cancers (especially colon and rectal). Vegetarian meals still remain inadvisable for growing children, pregnant women and elderly people.

The Montignac Method, perfectly compatible with a vegetarian approach, advises the consumption of a number of carbohydrates (having a low glycemic index):

- whole wheat bread
- whole grain bread
- brown rice
- whole wheat or whole grain pasta
- lentils
- white and kidney beans
- peas and snow peas
- whole grains and products made from them
- fresh and oleaginous fruits
- sugar-free marmalade
- soy and products made from it
- chocolate rich in cacao

Thus we can base the seven breakfasts of the week on fiber-rich bread or sugar-free cereal with a skim or chocolate – if necessary – dairy product. The Method also recommends making dinners based on good carbohydrates at least three times a week. Vegetarians can increase the frequency of this type of meal.

The main dish should be chosen from among the following suggestions:
- whole grain rice with tomato sauce,
- whole wheat or whole grain pasta with a basil, tomato, or mushroom sauce,
- lentils with onions,
- a combination of red and white beans
- peas
- chickpeas
- couscous made from whole semolina
- soy-based products
- grain-based products (whole wheat crepes)
- seaweed

As needed, these dishes can be embellished with vegetable soup, raw vegetables or a salad, and you can finish the meal with a dairy product, skim or whole, like cottage cheese or yogurt. Finally, let us stress that following a vegan diet in which dairy products and eggs are excluded in order to eat only foods of vegetable origin causes deficiencies. Doing so is <u>dangerous</u>.

Appendix III

FOR WOMEN WHO HAVE TROUBLE LOSING WEIGHT

Ask yourself if your present weight is not, in fact, your ideal weight. Some people want to reach an abnormally low weight for their frame size. The weight you were able to reach several years ago is not necessarily the correct current weight reference. Set yourself a realistic goal.

Perhaps you are making nutritional errors:

- The Montignac Method recommends eating at least three carbohydrate-rich meals based on whole-grain foods (pasta, rice or semolina) or legumes (lentils, white and kidney beans and chickpeas) each week among lunches and dinners. Are you following this recommendation?

- You need a sufficient amount of protein (60-90g per day, according to your weight). Some people do not follow this recommendation, and that can affect weight loss.

Do you consistently eat dairy products at each of your three meals? They contain a significant amount of protein and can even be enjoyed fat free.

- Is it possible that you are still caught in the low-calorie trap and eating almost nothing? **Losing weight does not mean eating less, but eating better.**
- Of course you are making good nutritional choices during meals, but maybe you are still snacking between meals or drinking alcohol. Doing so compromises weight loss.

Diet is not everything.

Of course good eating habits remain indispensable if you hope to lose weight, but that is not enough. Other factors can be involved:

- Unbalanced hormones in women (excess estrogen) can disturb weight loss (ask your doctor's opinion).
- The effects of stress can disturb your weight loss. If you are nervous, grieving or anxious, the body secretes chemical substances that can prevent weight loss. Learn to manage your stress with relaxation (sophrology) or yoga.
- An anomaly in the functioning of your thyroid (past or present) can prevent weight loss. Even if you have been treated and your body is well balanced, losing weight will always be a bit more difficult for you.
- A number of medicines can slow down weight loss: tranquilizers, anxiolytics, hypnotics, certain anti-depressants, lithium, cortisone, beta blockers, sweetened fortifiers and sometimes certain poorly adapted hormonal treatments for menopause (ask your doctor).

Do not confuse excess weight with cellulite or water retention. The treatments are not the same.

Appendix IV

HOW DO I MAKE SURE I GET ENOUGH PROTEIN?

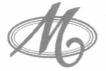

Healthy people of normal build should consume enough protein to make up for what is lost during cell renewal and to prevent the risk of muscle deterioration. That amount is around 1g for 2 lb. of body weight per day. (The minimum under which renewal is no longer assured is officially 0.80g).

That means that for a person weighing 155 pounds, the recommended daily intake of protein must be around 70g. When you begin a weight loss plan, your protein intake must be increased (from 1.3-1.5g per 2 lb. of body weight per day) for two reasons:

- First, all weight loss leads to some muscle loss. To limit this loss and avoid weakening the body (which is what happens when you follow low-calorie diets) it is best to consume more protein than what is needed for normal cell renewal.

- Second, it has been shown that a larger protein intake could be a supplementary aid in weight loss. Proteins cause you to feel fuller, contributing to naturally limiting your appetite. And, the digestion of proteins leads to greater energy use (thermogenesis).

But in order to eliminate the waste left over from protein metabolism, it is indispensable to drink plenty of liquids throughout the day: 1.5-2 quarts.

Increasing your protein intake complements the success of your weight loss program. Just the same, individuals who suffer from kidney problems should abstain from raising their protein ration without medical opinion. If your body is resistant to weight loss, you should verify that your daily protein intake is sufficient.

ANIMAL PROTEIN		VEGETABLE PROTEIN	
beef	20g	soy beans	35g
veal	20g	wheat germ	25g
pork	17g	oatmeal	13g
mutton	15g	rye germ	13g
cooked ham	18g	wheat germ	12g
smoked ham	15g	barley germ	10g
black pudding	24g	corn	9g
sausage	25g	whole wheat bread	9g
chicken	20g	whole wheat pasta	8g
one egg	6g	white beans	8g
fish	30g	lentils	8g
muenster	35g	chickpeas	8g
gruyère	35g	kidney beans	8g
brie	20g	white bread	7g
camembert	20g	wheat semolina	5g
cottage cheese	9g	white pasta	3g
yogurt	5g	brown rice	7g
milk	3.5g	white rice	6g
mussels	20g	granola	9g
shrimp	25g	tofu	13g
		soy flour	45g
		soy milk	4g
		soy germ	4g

Appendix V

TESTIMONIES ON THE EFFICACY OF THE MONTIGNAC METHOD: SUCCESSFUL STUDIES

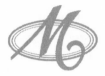

Since the first books on the Montignac Method were published in 1986/87, even before scientific studies were conducted by open-minded nutritionists curious to verify the benefits of our principles, hundreds of thousands of readers regulated their weight problems for good, thanks to the Method. The huge amount of mail we received from French and foreign readers, as well as the positive testimony of hundreds of doctors who have prescribed the Method, have always encouraged us to continue our research.

If we look at these testimonies, we can come to the following conclusions: around 85% of the people who apply the principles of the Method according to our recommendations obtain substantial long-term results. A minority encounters resistance to weight loss for very particular reasons, such as those touched on in Appendix III.

All those who successfully practice the Method declare that following it is simple, easy, and even agreeable, to the point of rediscovering the pleasure of eating. They have understood that the Method is not a diet but a new food philosophy. Some feel so good in Phase I that they do not even feel the need to go to Phase II.

All the testimonies agree on the point that they recognize that besides easily being able to stabilize weight loss, the change in eating habits according to the principle of the Method leads to:
- the disappearance of a certain number of gastrointestinal problems,
- better physical and intellectual shape (suppression of fatigue in general and sudden "slumps" in particular),
- a shorter and more refreshing sleep,
- better resistance to sickness, probably due to a diet that is richer in micronutrients (vitamins, minerals, and trace elements).

SCIENTIFIC STUDIES ON THE METHOD
The 1994 French Centre d'Etudes et d'Information des Vitamines' (CEIV) Study:

The study's goal was not to examine the efficacy of the Montignac Method, but to assess its nutritional makeup, especially its vitamin content. The study of nutritional journals kept by patients who were following the Method and of meals proposed in the books led to the following nutritional makeup:

Proteins	29.3%
Carbohydrates	39.5%
Fats	31.2%, including 332 mg of cholesterol per day
Fiber	24.4g per day
Phosphorus	1431 mg per day
Magnesium	447

Calcium		1110
Iron		18.6
Sodium		1643
Potassium		3465
Vitamin	C	198mg
	B1	2.6mg
	B2	3.1mg
	B6	1.8
	PP	24
	E	10.1
	D	1.4microg
	A	2080microg or 6939IU
	B9	509microg
Beta carotene		6400microg

In total we observe that the Montignac Method is among the best of the weight loss Methods in terms of micronutrient intake (vitamins and minerals). In addition, and contrary to the dishonest allegations of the Method's opponents (especially Dr. Jacques Fricker), it does not lead to an excessive consumption of fats because the Method's 31.2% fat content is in accordance with official nutritional recommendations.

Studies by Drs. Caupin and Robert

In 1994, these two doctors of the Institut Vitalité Et Nutrition of Paris began an open moving study on 150 women from 18 to 68 years of age divided into three groups based on their BMI.[1]
32 women had a BMI less than 24
80 women had a BMI between 24 and 29
38 women had a BMI greater than 29

---

[1] See Chapter 12 for information on BMI (Body Mass Index).

Results at the end of four months:

BMI	Average weight loss	Percentage of lost weight	Drop in BMI	Percentage of drop in BMI
<24	-5.47 kg	-8.81%	-2.11	-9.2%
24-29	-8.71 kg	-11.86%	-3.24	-11.85%
30-40	-13.37 kg	-14.42%	-5.09	-14.55%

Results at the end of one year:

BMI	Average weight loss	Percentage of lost weight	Drop in BMI	Percentage of drop in BMI
<24	-4.38 kg	-6.74%	-1.76	-7.9%
24-29	-8.14 kg	-10.41%	-3.00	-10.9%
30-40	-18.46 kg	-19.77%	-6.96	-20.22%

All of these people knew the principles of the Montignac Method, either as a result of studying them in the author's publications or because they were informed by their doctor.

Commentaries:

- For the group whose BMI was less than 24, which corresponds to a normal build (for example, a woman measuring 1.65m [about 5'5"] tall and weighing 60 kg [about 132 lb.]: some women having this normal BMI still wanted to be thinner, despite the opinion of the practitioner.

As the above table shows:

At the end of four months, we not an average weight loss of about 5.5 kg (about 12 lb.).

At the end of a year, the body, doubtlessly "finding" the new weight uselessly low, gained back around 1 kg (about 2 lb.). Weight loss stops at around 4.5 kg (about 10 lb.).

- For the group whose BMI was between 24 and 29, which corresponds to a weight in excess of a few pounds, (for example, a woman measuring 1.65 m [5'5"] and weighing 70kg [about 155 lb.] has a BMI of 27):

In the study, these women lost an average of 8.7 kg (about 19 lb.) in four months, meaning they reached their ideal weight. At the end of one year, they had gained back less than 600g (about 1 lb.). The Montignac Method helped obtain the correct stabilization of a normal weight.

- For the group whose BMI was between 30 and 40, which corresponds to true obesity:

After four months, these obese women had lost an average of 13.4 kg (about 30 lb.). At the end of one year, the average weight loss was 18.5 kg (about 40 lb.).

We can then say that weight loss occurs, even if it happens more slowly as the body gets closer to its ideal weight.

Canadian study by Professors Dumesnil and Tremblay:

Professor Dumesnil, cardiologist at the Institute of Cardiology of Laval Hospital in Quebec, was heavy and could not lose weight. One of his colleagues at the hospital recommended the Montignac Method to him. After he had lost 21 kilos (about 46 lb.), his colleague, the nutritionist Professor Tremblay was so intrigued that in 1997 the two decided to begin a study in order

	Diet 1	Diet 2 (Montignac)	Diet 3
Proteins	15%	31%	16%
Fats	30%	32%	30%
Carbohydrates	55%	37%	54%

to better understand the active parameters of the Montignac Method. So the authors compared the effects of several diets in men of about 47 years old having a BMI of 28 and an average weight of 103 kilos (225 lb.). In the three diets, the participants could eat as much as they wanted. Group II (Montignac Method) only had access to carbohydrates having a very low glycemic index. The average divisions of the different nutritional contents of each of the groups that could make its choices haphazardly during the study were the following:

Diet 2, which applied the advice of the Montignac Method (carbohydrates having a very low glycemic index) provides the best reduction of hunger and the best satiety, compared to the two others. This is essentially because of the choice of carbohydrates with low glycemic indexes imposed on the participants, but may also be the result of a greater consumption of proteins (1.55g per kg of weight), even though this choice was optional.

If we compare the relative percentage of change in weight:

Diet 1 (which corresponds to the nutritional advice of "classical dietetics") caused a 0.2% weight gain. The subject gained weight.

Diet 3 (which has the same calorie content as diet 2, but a different nutritional content, "classical" as we would say) only causes a 1.7% weight loss.

The best result is obtained with diet 2 (the Montignac Method) with an average weight loss of 2.4% of the initial weight (about 3.2 kg or 6.5 lb. in one week for a subject weighing 102 kg or 225 lb.). In addition, among the three diets, No.2 (Montignac) was the only one to show highly significant improvement in the domain of cardiovascular risk. However, as this will be newly published by Professor Dumesnil, the final figures are not yet available.

This study was officially presented (after a selection) at the Eighth International Congress on obesity in Paris in August 1998, where it attracted particular attention.

In the months following the publication of this book, the results of two large epidemological studies conducted in the US over twelve years by Professor Walter Willett of Harvard University's School of Public Health will be officially published. These studies 100% validate all the scientific hypotheses made by the Montignac Method since 1987. They show, in effect, that it is the consumption of high glycemic-index carbohydrates that is at the origin of the prevalence of obesity, diabetes, cardiovascular diseases and even cancer of our modern society. Professor Willett is particularly critical of his nutritionist colleagues by affirming that it is precisely their nutritional recommendations consisting of eating more carbohydrates and fewer fats that are largely responsible for the prevalence of obesity in the American population.

APPENDIX VI

Appendix VI

CULINARY PREPARATIONS AND DIVERSE RECIPES

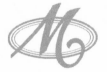

The object of this book is not to give you an impressive list of recipes to go with its contents. For that, there are a number of Montignac recipe books, which will find their way to your bookstore soon.

But if you have understood the basic dietary principles that you must adopt in order to attain the goal you set for yourself, you should be able to make your recipes yourself, or at least be able to modify those that you already know.

The respect of the principles of the Montignac Method is therefore translated into both the culinary domain and that of food choices in the following way:

1st – Elimination of all carbohydrates (sugar, starch, etc.) that have negative nutritional potential (high glycemic indexes), especially:

- sugar (saccharose)
- white flour
- potatoes
- cooked carrots
- corn
- white rice (except Basmati)
- noodles, macaroni and ravioli

2nd – On the other hand, give preference to all carbohydrates with positive nutritional potential:

- lentils
- dried beans
- peas
- chickpeas
- all green vegetables (lettuce, broccoli, cabbage, green beans, spinach, eggplant, peppers, tomatoes, zucchini, etc.)
- all whole grains (unrefined flours)
- fruit

3rd – Elimination of bad fats.

Avoid using:
- melted butter
- refined oils
- palm oil
- lard
- margarine

Instead use:
- olive oil
- goose fat

- duck fat
- sunflower oil
- nut oil or rapeseed oil

4th -- Elimination of any kind of breadcrumbs (breading)

5th – Opt for fish (fat) rather than meat (except poultry).

6th – Eliminate all cooking at high temperatures, especially frying.

These nutritional principles are applied in the following way in culinary practice:

<u>Appetizers:</u> Avoid all dishes made from white flour and butter: puff pastries, quiche, crepes, toast, croutons, etc.

<u>Main dishes:</u> Avoid frying especially with breading. If necessary, replace this with Parmesan.
- Avoid all sauces containing butter and especially wheat flour.
- Lentil and chickpea flours are welcome.
- The side dishes for fish, meat and poultry must conform to points one and two. Any kind of cheese is welcome (fresh, fermented, etc.), as well as yogurt (sugar/sweet flavor free).

<u>Desserts:</u> They must not contain flour, butter, or sugar. They should be made with fruit mousses, eggs, fresh cheese, almond flour, hazel nuts, or dark chocolate with minimum 70% dark cacao and fructose (see recipes). Wine may be used in the preparations.

Salad of Avacados and Artichoke Bottoms with Crab

Preparation: 15 minutes
Cooking time: 5 minutes

SERVES 6-8:

1 large (11 oz.) tin of crab
2 avocados
4 artichokes
2 sticks celery
1 lettuce
2 lemons

For the dressing:
1 egg yolk
Sunflower oil
1/2 tablespoon low-fat sour cream
2 tablespoons chopped parsley
Salt, pepper

Wash and drain the lettuce. Trim the artichoke bottoms, remove the hairy choke and dip in lemon juice to prevent discoloration. Cut into strips and cook in boiling salted water for 5 minutes. Once cooked, place under cold running water and drain.

Remove the stones from the avocados and shape the flesh into little balls, using a melon-baller. Pour lemon juice over them to prevent discoloration.

Cut the celery sticks into small pieces and mingle all the salad ingredients with the crab.

Make a mayonaise, using sunflower oil, and add the a sour cream and the chopped parsley. Season with salt en pepper.
Serve the crab salad dressed with the mayonaise.

Greek-Style Scampi

Preparation: 15 *minutes*
Cooking time: 40 *minutes*

SERVES 6-8:

36 to 48 scampi
(Dublin Bay prawns, langoustines)

2 large tins skinned tomatoes
4 oz. feta cheese
2 chopped onions
1 large bunch parsley
1 cup dry white wine
2 tablespoons olive oil
1 teaspoon oregano
Salt, pepper

Shell the scampi, retaining only the tail. Rinse under running water and dry on kitchen paper.

Fry the chopped onions on a low heat in the olive oil. Add the tinned tomatoes, drained, the white wine, half the chopped parsley, the oregano and the salt and pepper.

Simmer, uncovered, until the liquid had evaporated. Place the scampi in a pan with the rest of the olive oil. When golden brown, drain.

Add to the tomatoes little by little and sprinkle with thinly sliced feta. Cook for 5 minutes, stirring very gently.

Serve decorated with chopped parsley.

Filets of Sole
with an Aubergine Puree

Preparation: 20 *minutes*
Cooking time: 30 *minutes*

SERVES 4:

4 sole fillets (5 oz. each)
1-2 tablespoons of court-bouillon
2 lb. aubergines
1 lemon
6 tablespoons olive oil
4 leaves basil
Salt, pepper

Grill the aubergines for 30 minutes, turning during this time, so that all the skin is well done (almost burnt).

Remove the skin and seeds and blend the flesh with the olive oil, lemon juice, basil, salt and pepper.

Arrange the sole fillets in an ovenproof dish. Pour the court-bouillon over and cook in a hot oven (400°F) for 5 to 7 minutes.

Arrange the sole fillets on a warmed serving dish with the aubergine purée around them.

Suggestions:
Spinach makes a suitable additional accompaniment.

Parcels of Salmon Fillet
with a Puree of Green Peppers

Preparation: 15 minutes
Cooking time: 45 minutes

SERVES 4:

4 salmon fillets (5 oz. each)
2 new onions
2 tablespoons low-fat sour cream
4-5 green peppers
1 lemon
5 tablespoons dry white wine
Salt, pepper

Wrap the peppers in cooking foil and bake in a hot oven (500°F) for 45 minutes.

Meanwhile, cook the slices onions in the white wine until it has evaporated.

Season the fish with salt and pepper and squeeze a few drops of lemon over it. Wrap immediately in envolopes of cooking foil. Bake in a hot oven (500°F) for 10 minutes.

Peel the peppers, cut them in half and blend with the onions and sour cream. Adjust the seasoning and serve the salmon surrounded by the purée of peppers.

Duck with Artichokes and Olives

Preparation: 25 minutes
Cooking time: 50 minutes

SERVES 4:

1 oven-ready duck (2¹/₂-3¹/₂ lb.)
4 skinned tomatoes
8 cooked artichoke bottoms
20 black olives
3 tablespoons olive oil
6 sliced shallots
1 (9 oz.) tin mushrooms
1 tablespoon low-fat sour cream
1 bay leaf, thyme, basil
Salt, pepper
1 clove garlic

Cut the tomatoes in quarters, remove the seeds and cut into stripes. Cut the artichokes into thick slices. Stone the olives and slice in half.

Joint the duck and brown in olive oil on a high heat. Add the tomatoes, sliced shallots and garlic and season with salt and pepper. Blend the mushrooms to a purée and add a tablespoon of low-fat sour cream.

Add the mushroom purée, bay leaf and slices of artichoke.

Cover and cook over a medium heat for 50 minutes. 2 minutes from the end of the cooking time, add the black olives.

Remove the bay leaf before serving.

Duck Breasts in Green Pepper Sauce

Preparation: 25 minutes
Cooking time: 20 minutes

SERVES 4:

4 duck breasts
1/2 lb. mushrooms
1 lemon
1/2 cup wine
1 onion
1 bay leaf
30 green peppercorns
1 tablespoon olive or sunflower oil

Slice the onions and soften in 1 tablespoon olive (or sunflower) oil. Add the red wine. Leave on a high heat until the liquid had almost completely evaporated.

Add 1 glass of water, the bay leaf and green pepper and cook for 15 minutes.

Trim and wash the mushrooms and cook whole in water with the lemon juice for 5 minutes. Blend to a purée, season with salt and add the <u>butter</u>. Strain the sauce through a sieve and return to a low heat to reduce. Add the mushroom purée.

Cook the duck breasts in a non-stick frying pan with no added fat or oil. Allow 4 minutes each side on a medium heat.

The duck breasts can be sliced into long, thin strips. Serve covered with the sauce.

Turkey Thigh with Lentil Purée

Preparation: 15 minutes
Cooking time: 1 hour 15 minutes

SERVES 6:

1 turkey thigh (2 ½ lb. cut into pieces)
7 oz. smoked bacon (in a piece, not rashers)
1 onion spiked with a clove
2 shallots
1 clove garlic
2 tablespoons low-fat sour cream
1 lb. green lentils
1 bouquet garni (thyme, rosemary, bay)
A few sprigs parsley
1 tablespoon olive oil
Salt, pepper

Soak the lentils in cold water for 12 hours. Dice the bacon and fry in a flame-proof casserole in 1 tablespoon of olive oil, with the sliced shallots.

When the shallots are golden, remove from the casserole and replace with the pieces of turkey. Fry these too until golden brown. Then return the bacon and shallots to the casserole and add the crushed garlic, the bouquet garni, salt, pepper and three cups of water. Simmer on a low heat for 1 hour 15 minutes.

Meanwhile, drain the lentils and cook for 45 minutes on a low heat, in salted (initially cold) water, together with the onion spiked with a clove, pepper and a few bay leaves.

Drain the lentils and put them through the blender, adding a little of the cooking water. Strain through a sieve and add the sour cream.

Serve the pieces of turkey accompanied by the lentil purée.

Stuffed Tomatoes

(Also works for eggplant, zucchini, green peppers, etc.)

SERVES 4-5:

6 good-sized tomatoes
1 lb. ground sausage
3/4 lb. mushrooms
1 onion
2 tbsp. fat-free sour cream
salt and pepper

Garlic and parsley optional.

Brown ground sausage; add salt and pepper to taste. Chop the onion, and purée in the blender.

Do the same with the mushrooms after washing them.

Combine the onion and mushrooms and sauté them in a little olive oil over low heat. Lightly salt.

Cut the tomatoes in half crosswise. Place them in a baking dish lightly greased with olive oil, and bake in a hot oven for 30 minutes.

Thoroughly mix together the ground sausage, 2/3 of the onion and mushroom purée, and the sour cream.

Evenly spread the mixture over the tomatoes after they have finished baking.

Use the last 1/3 of the onion and mushroom purée to sprinkle over the top of the tomatoes, as you would do with breadcrumbs. If you wish, you can add finely chopped garlic and parsley.

Bake in a hot oven (350-375°) for 30-40 minutes.

It is possible to broil the tomatoes by placing the baking dish in the middle of the oven to avoid burning.

Wholewheat Spaghetti Carbonara

Preparation: 5 minutes
Cooking time: 5 to 14 minutes

SERVES 4:

1 lb. wholewheat spaghetti (fresh or dried)
8 rashers lean bacon
1/2 cup sour cream
4 eggs
3 oz. grated parmesan
Salt, pepper

Cook the spaghetti in boiling salted water for 3 minutes if fresh or 6/7 minutes if dried. Drain and keep warm.

Cut the bacon into small pieces and fry for a few minutes on a high heat.

Remove half the fat in the pan, then add the cream and reduce for a few minutes.

Remove from the heat and add the lightly beaten eggs and grated parmesan. Season with salt and pepper, and keep warm.

Serve the pasta at once, with the carbonara sauce poured over.

Suggestions:
Can also be accompanied by a basil sauce or mushroom purée.

Chili Con Carne

Preparation: 30 minutes
Cooking time: 3 hours

SERVES 6:

2¼ lb. minced beef
11 oz. red kidney beans
3 onions
1 green pepper
2 cloves garlic
2¼ lb. tinned tomatoes
½ cup olive oil
2 Cayenne (finger) peppers
1 teaspoon ground cumin
4 cups chicken stock
1 teaspoon paprika

Soak the red kidney beans in cold water for 12 hours. Drain, cover with cold water, bring to the boil and cook on a medium heat for 1 hour. Half-way through cooking, add salt and skim. When the beans are done, drain and set on one side.

On a high heat, fry the minced beef in a flame-proof casserole in 3 tablespoons olive oil. Season with salt and paprika. Simmer for 10 minutes. Remove the meat and set on one side.

Wash and dice the green pepper and fry on a low heat in the casserole in 2 tablespoons olive oil. Add the sliced onions and the crushed garlic. When the onions are translucent, add the Cayenne peppers and the cumin.

Return the meat to the casserole and pour in the chicken stock. Add the tomatoes and mingle the ingredients together. Cover and cook on a low heat for 40 minutes.

Then add the red kidney beans and replace over a low heat to cook, uncovered, for a further 30 minutes.

Add more stock during cooking if necessary.

Serve hot.

Oyster Omelette

Preparation: 15 minutes
Cooking time: 7 minutes

SERVES 4:

8 eggs
12 oysters (flat type)
2 tablespoons chopped flat-leaved parsley
A dash of saffron
2 tablespoons single cream
Salt, pepper
3 tablespoons sunflower oil

Open the oysters and remove them from their shells. Keep the liquid and filter it into a saucepan. Heat the liquid but do not allow to boil. Plunge the oysters in for 30 seconds. Remove and set aside to keep warm.

Lightly beat the eggs with 2 tablespoons of the cooking liquid, a dash of saffron, salt and pepper.

Cook the omelette in sunflower oil. When it is almost ready, place the oysters (drained on absorbent kitchen paper) in the centre.

Fold the omelette and serve right away.

Eggplant Au Gratin

SERVES 6:

4 to 5 very nice eggplants
1 lb. ground sausage
1 lb. Tomatoes
1/2 lb. grated Gruyere
olive oil
tarragon

Dice the eggplant. Sauté over low heat in one or two pans, lightly adding olive oil. Constantly stir, cooking uniformly. (You can also lightly steam the eggplant.)

When the eggplant has changed color, add salt and pepper, and put them in a large baking dish. Bake for 40 minutes at around 300°.

While you wait, completely reduce the tomatoes as in the previous recipe. Separately, cook the ground sausage, separating all the pieces.

When the eggplant is almost cooked, add the sausage and tomato sauce, stirring to create a uniform mixture.

Sprinkle the grated Gruyere and tarragon over the entire dish.

Put everything back into the oven on the center rack for 15 minutes.

The eggplant au gratin can make up the main course of the meal.

Caesar Salad

Preparation: 30 *minutes*
Cooking time: 10 *minutes*

SERVES 4:

1 head of romaine lettuce
4 to 5 garlic cloves, minced
10 finely sliced anchovy filets
3 egg yolks
the juice from $1/2$ lemon
2 tablespoons balsamic vinegar
2 teaspoons Dijon mustard
5 tablespoons olive oil
4 slices bacon
6 oz. shredded parmesan
salt and pepper
1 teaspoon Worcestershire sauce

Wash and drain the lettuce. Cut the leaves into about 2-in. pieces. Chill at least 1 hour before serving.

In blender, place garlic, anchovies, egg yolks, lemon juice, vinegar, Worcestershire sauce and mustard. Blend until thickened. Little by little, add olive oil. The dressing should be very creamy. Add salt and pepper, and chill 2 to 3 hours.

Fry bacon over low heat in a non-stick pan until it is a little dry. Allow to cool, then chop into very small pieces in food processor.

To serve, place lettuce on large plates. Evenly add dressing. Generously sprinkle with Parmesan. Finish by adding bacon bits.

Brown Rice with Tomatoes

SERVES 4:

2 lb. of tomatoes (or a large can of whole tomatoes)
3 to 4 large onions
1 cup brown rice
olive oil

Finely chop onions and sauté in a little olive oil. Reduce tomatoes in a large pan after having cut them into small pieces.

When the onions are nicely browned, mix them into the tomatoes.

Reduce everything well over very low heat until obtaining a slightly consistent sauce; season with salt, pepper, and Cayenne pepper.

Cook the rice according to the directions on the package, after having salted the cooking water as for ordinary rice. Serve everything, either already combined or separately.

The rice dish could make up a whole meal. Beforehand, serve a good vegetable soup.

Oysters Served Hot with Raw Ham

Preparation: 10 minutes
Cooking time: 18 minutes

SERVES 4:

4 dozen good-sized oysters
2 good-sized slices raw ham
2 shallots, finely chopped
7 oz. fresh mushrooms, sliced
1 tablespoon lemon juice
2 pinches celery salt
1/2 cup low-fat sour cream
2 tablespoons chopped parsley
Salt, pepper

Open the oysters and remove from their shells. Filter the liquid. Cut the ham into strips and fry on a high heat.

Add the liquid from the oysters, together with the shallots, the sliced mushrooms, lemon juice, salt, pepper and celery salt.

Simmer, covered, for 5 minutes. Uncover and simmer for a further 5 minutes to reduce the cooking liquid.

Add the oysters and bring to the boil. Finally stir in the cream, sprinkle with parsley and leave over the heat for a further minute, stirring all the time.

Serve at once on warmed plates.

Scallops served on a Bed of Leeks

Preparation: 10 minutes
Cooking time: 15 minutes

SERVES 4:

16 scallops
7 oz. leeks (white part only)
8 tablespoons olive oil
1 glass dry white wine
A few leaves tarragon

Clean the leeks and slice thickly. Fry on a low heat in 2 tablespoons olive oil, without browning. Add the white wine and simmer for 15 minutes.

In another pan, sauté the scallops in olive oil for 2 minutes each side. Season with salt, pepper and chopped tarragon.

Place the leeks on warmed individual plates. Arrange the scallops on top.

Season with pepper, and serve.

Frozen Strawberries with Sauce

SERVES 8-10:

1 lb. of strawberries
4 oz. fat-free sour cream
5 egg whites
2 tbsp. lemon juice
5-6 tsp. powdered artificial sweetener
or 3 tbsp. fructose

Purée the strawberries in the blender or with an electric beater. Beat the egg whites until firm.

Combine the strawberry purée, the egg whites, the sour cream and the artificial sweetener until you have an even mixture.

Add the lemon juice and pour the mixture into a pre-greased plastic mold.

Place this in the freezer for approximately 6-7 hours. Remove from freezer 1/2 hour before serving.

To remove from mold, place mold under warm water.

Serve with sauce, decorating the dish with strawberries cut in half.

To make sauce:

Mix 1/2 pint strawberries with 2 tbsp. powdered artificial sweetener and the juice from half of a lemon.

Bavarian Raspberries with their Sauce

SERVES 5-6:

1 lb. of raspberries
4 egg yolks
1 3/4 c. milk
6 tsp. powdered artificial sweetener or
3 tbsp. fructose
3 sheets of gelatin, or equivalent

Soak the sheets of gelatin in cold water.

In a saucepan, beat the egg yolks and add the milk. Cook over low heat and allow to thicken until the mixture coats the spatula. Remove from heat.

Purée the raspberries in a blender, and add the artificial sweetener. Drain the gelatin and dissolve it in the warm milk. Combine the raspberries and the milk.

Pour into a lightly greased plastic mold, and allow to set for at least 12 hours in the refrigerator.

Serve cold with the raspberry sauce.

To make sauce:

Purée 1/2 pint raspberries, adding the juice of 1 lemon and 1/2 tsp. artificial sweetener.

Chocolate Mousse

SERVES 6-8:

14 oz. quality dark chocolate (2 tablets)
with at least 70% cocoa
8 eggs
3 tbs. rum
1 orange
4 tsp. ground coffee
a pinch of salt

Break the chocolate into pieces and put into the saucepan. Make a half-cup of strong coffee or espresso and add to chocolate along with the rum. Melt the chocolate over very low heat, stirring with the spatula to keep the mixture smooth. If mixture is really too thick, add a little water. As soon as the chocolate is perfectly melted into a thick, very unctuous liquid, remove pan from heat.

While the chocolate is melting, grate the orange peel (only use the top part of the skin; the white pith is bitter), and add half to the chocolate mixture. Break the eggs, separating the whites from the yolks. Put them in two separate bowls. Beat the egg whites with a pinch of salt until stiff.

Pour the chocolate mixture into the bowl containing the yolks. Mix well until smooth and homogenous. Next add this to the whites, and mix well with the spatula. Make sure there are no unmixed pieces of chocolate or egg whites at the bottom of the bowl.

You can either leave the mousse in the mixing bowl or pour it into individual dishes. Before putting it in the refrigerator sprinkle the rest of the orange zest on top.

Make the mousse at least six hours prior to serving. Ideally, make it the night before.

Bitter Chocolate Cake

14 oz. bitter dark chocolate (2 tablets) with at least
70% dark cocoa
2 tbs. cognac
8 eggs
1 orange
4 tsp. instant coffee

Break the chocolate into pieces and put into saucepan. Make a half-cup strong coffee or espresso and add to chocolate with cognac. Melt chocolate over very low heat, stirring with spatula to obtain a smooth, creamy mixture. Once it is completely melted, remove from heat.

Break the eggs, separating the whites from the yolks. Beat the whites with a pinch of salt until they are stiff.

Pour the melted chocolate into the bowl containing the egg yolks. Mix well until smooth. Next, add this mixture to the whites and mix with the spatula. The mixture must be completely homogenous. Make sure that no unmixed egg whites or chocolate remain at the bottom of the bowl.

Pour this mousse into the cake pan greased with butter, or better yet, lined with waxed paper.

Put into oven preheated to 250°. Bake for just 8 minutes so that the cake stays soft in the middle.

Serve in slices, either as-is or accompanied by custard or a scoop of vanilla ice cream.

Appendix VII

MICHEL MONTIGNAC PRODUCTS "FOR NUTRITIONAL GASTRONOMY"

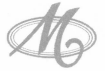

More than 120 products are available in order to eat healthy and remain gourmand every day. Michel Montignac has created a line of exclusive food products specifically designed to go with his Method. All are rich in fiber, without added sugar and made from whole-grain organic flour, and they all have a low glycemic index. In addition, they contain no additives, modified starches, or artificial colors.

Among these you will find specialties made with 100% real fruit, crackers and toast, shortbread cookies, chocolate containing high concentrations of cacao (72-85%), pasta, compotes, and sauces.

USEFUL ADDRESSES

CUSTOMER SERVICE AND POINTS OF SALE
for all information see
www.montignac-intl.com

BOUTIQUE MICHEL MONTIGNAC (New Diet SA)
14, rue de Maubeuge
75009 Paris
France
Telephone: 01 49 95 93 42

INSTITUT VITALITE ET NUTRITION
Medical advice, Education, Seminars
1, rue Robin
95880 ENGHIEN
France
Telephone: 01 39 83 18 39
Fax: 01 39 84 30 00

MONTIGNAC BOUTIQUE
160 Old Brompton Road
SW5 OBA London
UK

USA SERVICE AND INFORMATION
see
www.montignacusa.com

BIBLIOGRAPHY

PROTEINS:

APFELBAUM M., FORRAT C., NILLUS P. Diététique et nutrition Ed. Masson 1989

BOURRE J-M- De l'animal à l'assiette- Ed. Odile Jacob, 1993

BRINGER J., RICHARD JL, MIROUZE J. Evaluation de l'état nutritionnel protéique Rev. Prat. 1985,35,3,17-22

CHELTIEL J.C Protéines alimentaires - Ed, Tech et Doc Lavoisier, 1985

RUASSE JP Les composants de la matière vivante Ed. L'indispensable en nutrition 1988

RUASSE JP Des protides, pourquoi, combien? Ed. L'indispensable en nutrition 1987

CARBOHYDRATES:

ANDERSON JW - Hypocholesterolemic effects of oat and bean products - Am.J.Clin.Nutr., 1988, 48, 749-753

ANDERSON JW - Serum lipid response of hypercholesterolemic men to single and divided doses of canned beans Eur. J. Clin. Nutr., 1990, 51, 1013-1019.

AUBERT C.- L'assiette aux céréales - Ed. Terre vivante, 1991

BANTLE J.P, LAINE D.C. Post prandial glucose and insulin responses to meals containing different carbohydrates in normal and diabetic subjets New Engl. J. Med. 1983, 309,7-12

BIBLIOGRAPHY

BORNET F. Place des glucides simples et des produits amylacés dans l'alimentation des diabétiques en 1985.
Fondation RONAC.Paris

BROWN Coronary heart disease and the consumption of diet high in wheat and other grains.
Am.J. Clin. Nutr., 1985, 41 1163-1171

CALET C.- Les légumes secs, apport protidique, Cah. Nutr. Diet., 1992, XXVII, 2, 99-108

CHEW I. Application of glycemic index to mixed meals
Am. J. Clin- Nutr. 1988,47,53-56

CRAPO P.A. Plasma glucose and insulin responses to orally administered simple and complex carbohydrates
Diabetes 1976,25,741-747

CRAPO P.A. Post prandial plasma glucose and insulin response to different complex carbohydrates
Diabetes 1977,26,1178-1183

CRAPO P.A. Comparaison of serum glucose-insulin and glucagon responses to different types of carbohydrates in non insulin dependant diabetic patients Am J. Clin. Nutr. 1981, 34,84-90

DANQUECHIN-DORVAL E.Rôle de la phase gastrique de la digestion sur la biodisponibilité des hydrates de carbone et leurs effets métaboliques Journées de diabétologie de l'Hôtel-Dieu 1975

DESJEUX J.F. Glycémie, insuline et acides gras dans le plasma d'adolescents sains après ingestion de bananes
Med. et Nutr. 1982,18,2,127-130

FEWKES D.W. Sucrose-Science Progres 1971, 59. 25, 39

FITZ-HENRY A. In vitro and in vivo rates of carbohydrate digestion in Arboriginal bushfoods and contemporary Western foods.
(colloque 1982 de l'Université de Sydney)

GABREAU T, LEBLANC H. Les modifications de la vitesse d'absorption des glucides
Med. et Nutr. 1983, XIX, 6,447-449

GUILLAUSSEAU P.J, GUILLAUSSEAU-SCHOLER C. Effet hyperglycémiant des aliments Gaz. Med. Fr. 1989, 96, 30, 61-63

HEATON K.W. Particule size of wheat, maïze and oat test meals : effects on plasma glucose and insulin responses and on the rate
of starch digestion in vitro Am. J. Clin. Nutr. 1988,47,675-682

HODORA D. Glucides simples, glucides complexes et glucides indigestibles Gaz. Med. Fr. 1981, 88,37,5,255-259

JENKINS D.J.A. Glycemic index of foods : a physiological basis for carbohydrates exchange
Am. J ; Clin. Nutr. 1981, 34, 362-366

JENKINS D.J.A. Dietary carbohydrates and their glycemic responses J.A.M.A. 1984, 2, 388-391

JENKINS D. J.A. Wholemeal versus wholegrain breads: proportion of whole or cracked grains and the glycemic response
Br. Med. J 1988,297,958-960

JIAN R. La vidange d'un repas ordinaire chez l'homme : étude par la méthode radio-isotopique
Nouv. Presse Med. 1979, 8, 667-671

KERIN O'DEA Physical factor influencing post prandial glucose and insulin responses to starch
Am. J. Clin. Nutr. 1980, 33,760-765

MESSING B- Sucre et nutrition. Ed Doin, 1992

NOUROT J. Relationship between the rate of gastric emptying and glucose insulin responses to starchy food in young healty adults. Am. J. Clin. Nutr. 1988. 48, 1035-1040

NATHAN D. Ice-cream in the diet of insulin-dependant diabetic patients J.A.M.A. 1984, 251, 21, 2825-2827

NICOLAIDIS S. Mode d'action des substances de goût sucré sur le métabolisme et sur la prise alimentaire. Les sucres dans l'alimentation.
Cool. Sc. Fond. Fr. Nutr. 1981

O'DONNEL L.J.D. Size of flour particles and its relation to glycemia, imulinaemia and caloric disease.
Br. Med. J. 17 June 1984, 298,115-116

PICHARD P. Les céréales énergétiques - Ed. M.A., 1992

PIVETAUD J., PACCALIN J.
Mais mangez donc des légumineuses !
Diététique et Médecine, 1993, n°4, 149-153

REAVEN C. Effects of source of dietary carbohydrates on plasma glucose and insulin to test meals in normal subjects
Am. J. Clin. Nutr. 1980, 33, 1279-1283

ROUX E. Index glycémique Gaz. Med. Fr; 1988,95,18,77-78

RUASSE JP Des glucides, pourquoi, comment ?
Collection "L'indispensable en nutrition"

SCHLIENGER JL Signification d'une courbe d'hyperglycémie orale plate, comparaison avec un repas d'épreuve Nouv. Pr. Med. 1982, 52, 3856-3857

SCHWEITZER TF Nutrients excreted in ileostomy effluents after consumption of mixed diet with beans and potatoes, Eur. J. Clin. Nutr. 1990, 44, 567-575

SLAMA G. Correlation between the nature of amount of carbohydrates in intake and insulin delivery by the artificiel pancreas in 24 insulino-dependant diabetics
1981,30,1 01-105

SLAMA G. Sucrose taken during mixed meal has no additional hyperglyceamic action over isocaloric amounts of starch in well-controlled diabetics Lancet, 1984,122-124

SPRING B. Psychological effects of carbohydrates, J.Clin. Psychiatry, 1989, 50-5, suppl., 27-33

STACH J.K. Contribution à l'étude d'une diététique rationnelle du diabétique :rythme circadien de la tolérance au glucose, intérêt pain complet, intérêt du sorbitol. Thèse pour le doctorat en Médecine, Caen 1974

TORSDOTTIR I. - Gastric emptying and glycemic response following ingestion of mashed bean or potato flakes in composite meals

Am. J. Clin. Nutr. Diet, 1990 (sous presse en 1990, cité par Bornet in Cah.Nutr.Diet., 1990, XXV, 4, 254-264)

THORBURN A.W. The glyceemic index of food Med. J. Austr. May 26 th 1988 144, 580-582

VAGUE P. Influence comparée des différents glucides alimentaires sur la sécrétion hormonale. Les sucres dans l'alimentation, Collection Scientifique de la Fondation Française pour la Nutrition

LIPIDS:

BOURRE J.M-DURAND G. The importance of dietary linoleic acid in composition of nervous membranes.
Diet and life style, new technology De M.F.Mayol, 1988 John Libbey Eurotext Ldt p. 477-481

BOURRE J.M — Les bonnes graisses- Ed. Odile Jacob, 1991

DREON D.M. — The effects of polyinsatured fat versus monoinsatured fat on plasma lipoproteins JAMA, 1990, 263, 2462-2466

DYERBERG J. — Linolenic acid and eicosapentaenoic acid Lancet 26 Janvier 1980, p. 199

GUERGUEN L. — Interactions lipides-calcium alimentaires et biodisponibilité du calcium du fromage Cah. Nutr. Diet.,1992, XXVII, 5, 311-314

JACOTOT B. — Olive oil and the lipoprotein metabolism. Rev. Fr. des Corps Gras 1988,2,51-55

JACOTOT B. — L'huile d'olive, de la santé à la gastronomie- Ed. Artulen, 1993

KUSHI — Diet and 20 years mortality from coronary heart disease. The Ireland-Boston Diet-Heart study. New England J. of Medecine, 1985, 312 ; 811-818

LOUHERANTA A.M — Linoleic acid intake ans susceptibility of VLDL and LDL to oxidation in men Am.J.Clin. Nutr., 1996, 63, 698-703

LOUIS-SYLVESTRE J.   A propos de la consommation actuelle de lipides - Diétécom,1996

MAILLARD C.   Graisses grises Gazette Med. de Fr. 1989, 96, n° 22

MENSIK R.P.   Effect of dietary fatty acids on high density and low-density lipoprotein cholesterol levels in healthy

ODENT M.   Les acides gras essentiels - Ed. Jacques Ligier, 1990

RUASSE JP   Des lipides, pourquoi, comment ? Coll. L'Indispensable en Nutrition.

SAN JUAN P.M.F.   Study of isomeric trans-fatty acids content in the commercial Spanish foods
                            Int. J. of food Sc.&Nutr., 1996, 47, 399-403

TROISI R.   Trans-fatty acid intake in relation to serum lipid concentrations in adult men
                            Am.J.Clin.Nutr., 1992, 56, 1019-1024

VLES R.O.   Connaissances récentes sur les effets physiologiques des margarines riches en acide linoléique. Rev. Fr. des Corps Gras 1980, 3, 115-120

WILLETT W.C.   Intake of trans fatty acids and risk of coronary heart disease among women,
                            Lancet, 1993, 341, 581-585

FIBER:

« Concil Scientific Affairs » Fibres alimentaires et santé JAMA
                            1984,14,190,1037-1046

ANDERSON J. W.   Dietary fiber : diabetes and obesity Am. J. Gastroenterology 1986, 81, 898-906

BERNIER J.J.   Fibres alimentaires, motricité et absorption intestinale. Effets sur l'hperg1ycémie post-prandiale Journée de Diabétologie Hotel-Dieu 1979, 269-273

HABER G.B.   Depletion and disruption of dietary fibre. Effets on satiety plasma glucose and serum insulin.
                            Lancet 1977, 2, 679-682

HEATON K.W.   Food fiber as an obstacle to energy intake Lancet 1973, 2,1418-1421

HEATON K.W.   Dietary fiber in perspective Human Clin. Nutr. 1983,37c, 151-170

HOLT S.   Effect of gel fibre on gastric emptying and absorption of glucose and paracetamol
                            Lancet 1979, March 24, 636-639

JENKINS D.J.A.	Decrease in post-prandial insulin and glucose concentration by guar an pectin Ann. Int. Med. 1977. 86.20-33
JENKINS D.J.A.	Dietary fiber, fibre analogues and glucose - tolérance : importance of viscosity Br.Med. J. 1978, 1, 1392-1394
LAURENT B.	Etudes récentes concernant les fibres alimentaires Med. et Nutr. 1983, XIX, 2, 95-122
MONNIER L	Effets des fibres sur le métabolisme glucidique Cah. Nutr. Diet 1983, XVIII, 89-93
NAUSS K.M.	Dietary fat and fiber: relationship to caloric intake body growth and colon carcinogenesis Am. J Clin. Nutr. 1987, 45, 243-251
SAUTIER C.	Valeur alimentaire des algues spirulines chez l'homme Ann. Nutr. Alim 1975,29,517
SAUTIER C.	Les algues en alimentation humaine Cah. Nutr. Diet 1987.6,469-472

GENERAL POINTS ON CHOLESTEROL:

BASDEVANT A., TRAYNARD P.Y. Hypercholestérolémie, Symptômes 1988 n° 12

BRUCKERT E. Les dyslipidémies Impact Médecin, Dossier du Praticien n° 20, 1989

LUC G., DOUSTE-BLAZY P., FRUCHART JC Le cholestérol, d'ou vient-il ?
Comment Circule-t-il ? Ou va t-il ?
Rev. Prat 1989, 39, 12,1011-1017

POLONOWSKI J. Régulation de l'absorption intestinale du cholestérol Cahiers Nutr. Diet 1989,1,19-25

LIPIDS & CHOLESTEROL:

Consensus : Conference on lowering blood cholesterol to prevent heart disease JAMA 1985, 253, 2080-2090

BETTERIDGE DJ High density lipoprotein and coronary heart disease Brit. Med. J. 15 Avril 1989,974-975

DURAND G. and all Effets comparés d'huiles végétales et d'huiles de poisson sur le cholestérol du rat.
Med. et Nutr. 1985, XXI, N° 6,391-406

DYERBERG J. and all Eicosapentaenoic acid and prevention of thrombosis and atherosclerosis. Lancet 1978, 2, 117-119

ERNST E.,LE MIGNON D. Les acides gras omega 3 et l'artériosclérose CR de Ther. 1987, V, N°56,22-25

FIELD C. The influence of eggs upon plasma cholesterol levels Nutr. Rev. 1983,41, N°9,242-244

FOSSATI P., FERMON C. Huiles de poisson, intérêt nutritionnel et prévention de l'athéromatose
Nouv. Presse. Med. 1988, VIII, 1-7

de GENNES J.L, TURPING. TRFFERT J. Correction thérapeutique des hyperlipidémies idiopathiques héréditaires. Bilan d'une consultation Consultation de diététique standardisée Nouv. Presse Med. 1973,2,2457-2464

GRUNDY M.A. Comparaison of monosatured fatty acids and carbohydrates for lowering plasma cholesterol
N. Engl. J. Med. 1986,314,745-749

HAY C.R.M. Effect of fish oil on platelet kinetics in patients with ischaemic heart disease The Lancet 5 Juin 1982,12691272

KRUMHOUT D., BOSSCHIETER E.B., LEZENNE-COULANDER C.
The inverse relation between fish consumption and 20 year mortality from coronary heart disease
New. Engl. J. Med. 1985, 312,1205-1209

LEAF A, WEBERPC Cardiovascular effects of n-3 fatty acides New Engl. J. Med. 1988,318,549-557

LEMARCHAL P. Les acides gras polyinsaturés en Oméga 3. Cah. Nutr. Diet. 1985, XX, 2,97-102

MARINIER E. Place des acides gras polyinsaturés de la famille n-3 dans le traitement des dysloprotéinémies
Med. Dig. Nutr. 1986,53,14-16

MARWICK C. What to do about dietary saturated fats ? JAMA 1989,262,453

PHILLIPSON and all Reduction of plasma lipids, lipoproteins and apoproteins by dietary fish oils in patients with hypertriglyceridemia
New Engl.J.Med 1985, 312, 1210-1216

PICLET G. Le poisson, aliment, composition, intérêt nutritionnel
Cah. Nutr. Diet 1987, XXII 317-336

THORNGREN M. Effects of 11 week increase in dietary eicosapentaenoïc acid on bleeding time, lipids and platelet aggregation Lancet 28 Nov. 1981,1190-11

TURPIN G. Régimes et médicaments abaissant la cholestérolémie Rev. du Prat. 1989,39, 12, 1024-1029

VLES R.O. Les acides gras essentiels en physiologie cardio-vasculaire Ann. Nutr. Alim. 1980,34,255-264

WOODCOCK B.E. Beneficial effect of fish oil on blood viscosity in peripheral vascular disease
Br. Med. J. Vol 288 du 25 février 1984, p. 592-594

DIETARY FIBER & HYPERCHOLESTEROLEMIA:

ANDERSON J.W. Dietary fiber lipids and atherosclerosis Am. J. Cardiol. 1987, 60,17-22

GIRAULT A. Effets bénéfiques de la consommation de pommes sur le métabolisme lipidique chez l'homme.
Entretiens de Bichat 28 Septembre 1988

LEMONNIER D., DOUCET C, FLAMENT C. Effet du son et de la pectine sur les lipides sériques du rat
Cah. Nutr. Diet. 1983. XVII, 2, 97

RAUTUREAU J., COSTE T., KARSENTI P. Effets des fibres alimentaires sur le métabolisme du cholestérol
Cah. Nutr. Diet 1983, XVIII, 2,84-88

SABLE-AMPLIS R, SICART R., BARON A. Influence des fibres de pomme sur le taux d'esters de cholestérol du foie, de l'intestin et de l'aorte Cah. Nutr. Diet 1983 XVII, 2, 97

TAGLIAFFERRO V. and all Moderate guar-gum addition to usual diet improves peripheral sensibility to insulin and lipaemic profile in NIDDM Diabète et Métabolisme 1985, 11, 380-385

TOGNARELLI M. Guar-pasta: a new diet for obese subjects Acta Diabet. Lat. 1986,23,77

TROWELL H. Dietary fiber and coronary heart disease Europ. J. Clin. Biol. Res. 1972,17,345

VAHOUNY G.U. Dietary fiber lipid metabolism and atherosclerosis Fed. Proc. 1982, 41, 2801-2806

ZAVOLAL JH. Effets hypolipémiques d'aliments contenant du caroube Am. J. Clin. Nutr. 1983,38,285-294

VITAMINS, TRACE ELEMENTS & HYPERCHOLESTEROLEMIA:

1. Vitamin E

CAREW T.E. Antiatherogenic effect of probucol unrelated to ist hypocholesterolemic effect P.N.A.S.
USA June 1984, Vol. 84 p 7725-7729

FRUCHART JC Influence de la qualité des LDL sur leur métabolisme et leur arthérogénicité (inédit)

JURGENS G. Modification of human serum LDL by oxydation Chemistry and Physics of lipids 1987,45,315-336

STREINBRECHER V.P. Modifications of LDL by endothelial cells involves lipid peroxydation P.NA.S.
USA June 1984, Vol. 81, 3883-3887

2. Selenium

LUOMA P.V. Serum selenium, glutathione peroxidase, lipids, and human liver microsomal enzyme activity
Biological Trace Element Research 1985, 8, 2,113-121

MITCINSON MJ. Possible role of deficiency of selenium and vitamin E in atherosclerosis J. Clin. Pathol. 1984, 37,7-837

SALONEN J.T. Serum fatty acids,apolipoproteins, selenium and vitamin antioxydants and risk of death from coronary
artery disease Am J. Cardiol. 1985, 56,4,226-231

3. Chromium

ABRAHAM A.S. The effect of chromium established atherosclerotic plaques in rabbits Am. J. Clin. Nutr. 1980.33,2294-2298

GORDON T. High density lipoprotein as a protective factor against coronary heart disease
The Framingham study Am. J. Med. 1977, 62, 707

OFFENBACHER EG Effect of chromium-rich yeast on glucose tolerance a blood lipids in elderly subjects Diabetes 1980, 29,919-925

COFFEE & HYPERCHOLESTEROLEMIA:

ARNESEN E. Coffee and serum cholesterol Br. Med. J. 1984,288,1960

HERBERT P.N. Caffeine does not affect lipoprotein metabolism Clin. Res. 1987, 35, 578A

HILL C. Coffee consumption and cholesterol concentration Letter to editor Br. Med. J. 1985, 290, 1590

THELLE D.S. Coffe and cholesterol in epidemiological and experimental studies Atherosclerosis 1987, 67, 97-103

THELLE D.S. The Tromso Heart Study. Does coffee raise serum cholesterol ? N. Engl. J. Med. 1983, 308, 1454-1457

GENERAL POINTS ON OBESITY:

ADRIAN F. Divergent trends in obesity and fat intake pattern : the American paradox Am.J.Med., 1997, 102, 259-264

ASTIER-DUMAS M. Densité calorique, densité nutritionnelle, repères pour le choix des aliments Med. Nutr. 1984, XX, 4, 229-234

BOUCHARD C. Génétique et métabolisme énergétique chez l'homme. In Forum Lavoisier, Paris, 1989

BELLISLE F. Obesity and food intake in children : evidence for a role of metabolic and/or behavioral daily rythms
Appetite 1988,11,111-118

BROWNELL KD. The effects of repeated cycles of weight loss and regain in rats Phys. Behaviour 1986, 38,459-464

FRICKER J., APFELBAUM M.- Le métabolisme de l'obésité- La Recherche, 1989, 20, 207, 200-208

HERAUD G. Densité nutritionnelle des aliments Gaz. Med. FR. 1988, 95,13, 39-42

HILLS A.P., WAHLQUIST M.L . - Exercice and obesity - Ed.Smith-Gordon, 1994

LEIBEL RJ. Diminished energy requirements in reduced obese persons Metabolism 1984, 33,164-170

LOUIS-SYLVESTRE J. Consommation d'un plat allégé et répercussion sur la prise alimentaire totale. Le Généraliste, 1979, 1083

RIETVELD W.J. L'horloge biologique. Revue de nutrition, Diétécom 1991, 80

ROLLAND-CACHERA M.F., BELLISLE F. No correlation beetween adiposity and food intake : why are working class children fatter ? Am. J. Clin. Nutr. 1986, 44, 779-787

ROLAND-CACHERA M.F., DEHEEGER M. Adiposity and food intake in young children : the environmental challenge to individual susceptibility Br. Med. J. 1988, 296,1037-1038

ROLLAND-CACHERA M.F. la France est-elle privilégiée par rapport aux autres pays développés ? 1ère journées alimentation, kilos, santé, 1997

RUASSE J.P Des calories, pourquoi ? Combien ? Coll - L'indispensable en Nutrition 1987

RUASSE J.P. L'approche homéopathique du traitement des obésités Paris 1988

SPITZER L., RODIN J. Human eating behavior : a critical review of studi in normal weight and overweight individuals
Appetite 1981,2,293

LOUIS-SYLVESTRE J. Poids accordéon : de plus en plus difficile à perdre Le Gén. 1989,1087,18-20

DIETARY HABITS:

HERCBERG S. Apports nutritionnels d'un échantillon représentatif de la population du Val de Marne. Rev . Epidem. et Santé Publ., 1991, 39

MARCOCCHIN N. Comportement alimentaire en Lorraine in Précis de nutrition et diététique, fasc.10, Pub. Ardix Médical

RIGAUD D. et coll. Enquête de consommation alimentaire I- Energie et macronutriments Cah. Nutr. Diet., 1997, 32, 6, 379-389

INSULIN:

BASDEVANT A. Influence de la distribution de la masse grasse sur le risque vasculaire La Presse Médicale 1987,16,4

CLARK M.G. Obesity with insulin resistance. Experimental insights Lancet 1983, 2, 1236-1240

DANGUIR J. Infusion of insulin causes relative increase of slow wave sleep in rats. Brain Research, 1984, 306, 97-103

FROMAN L.A. Effect of vagotomy and vagal stimulation on insulin secretion Diabetes 1967,16,443-448

GROSS P.De l'obésité au diabète L'actualité diabétologique.N° 13, P. 1-9

GUY-GRAND B.   Variation des acides gras libres plasmatiques au cours des hyperglycémies provoquées par voie orale
Journées de Diabétologie de l'Hôtel-Dieu 1968, p 319

GUY-GRAND B.   Rôle éventuel du tissu adipeux dans l'insulino-résistance
Journées de Diabétologie de l'Hôtel-Dieu 1972, 81-92

JEANRENAUD B. Dysfonctionnement du système nerveux. Obésité et résistance à l'insuline
M/S Médecine-Science 1987,3,403-410

JEANRENAUD B Insulin and obesity Diabetologia, 1979,17,135-138

KOLTERMAN O.G Mechanisms of imulin resistance in human obesity. Evidence for receptor and post-receptor effects:
J. Clin. Invest. 1980,65,1272-1284

LAMBERT A.F- Enhancement by caffeine of glucagon-inducet and tolbutamide induced insulin release trom isolated foetal pancreatic tissue Lancet, 1967,1,1-19-819-820

LAMBERT A.E Organocultures de pancréas foetal de rat: étude morphologique et libération d'insuline in vitro
Journées de Diabétologie de l'Hôtel-Dieu 1969,115-129

LARSON B. Abdominal adipose tissue distribution, obesity and risk of cardio-vascular disease and death
Br. Med. J. 1984,288,1401-1404

LE MARCHAND-BRUSTEL Y. Résistance à l'insuline dans l'obésité M/S Médecine-Sciences 1987.3,394-402

LINQUETTE C. Précis d'endocrinologie Ed. Masson 1973, P 658-666

LOUIS-SYLVESTRE J. La phase céphalique de sécrétion d'insuline Diabète et métabolisme 1987,13,63-73

MARKS V. Action de différents stimuli sur l'insulinosécrétion humaine : influence du tractus gastro-intestinal
Journées de Diabétologie de l'Hôtel-Dieu 1969,179-190

MARLISSE E.B. Système nerveux central et glycorégulation Journées de Diabétologie de l'Hôtel-Dieu 1975, 7-21

MEYLAN M. Metabolic factors in insulin resistance in human obesity Metabolism 1987,36,256-261

BIBLIOGRAPHY

WOODS S.C. Interaction entre l'insulinosécrétion et le système nerveux central
Journées de Diabétologie de l'Hôtel-Dieu 1983

DIABETICS:

American Diabetes Association : clinical practice recommendations, Diabetes Care,
1995, 18, suppl.1, 16-19

ANDERSEN E.- Effect of rice-rich versus a potato-rich diet on glucose, lipoprotein
and cholesterol metabolism in noninsulindependent diabetics Am.J.Clin., Nutr., 1984,
39, 598-606

BORNET F.- Insulinemic and glycemic indexes of six starch-rich foods taken alone
and in a mixed meal by type 2 diabetic
Am. J. Clin. Nutr., 1987, 45, 588-595

BORNET F. Technologie des amidons, digestibilité et effets métaboliques- Cah. Nutr.
Diet., 1992, 27, 170-178

BRAND-MILLER J.C., - Importance of glycemic index in diabetes. Am. J Clin. Nutr.,
1994, 59 suppl., 747 S-752 S

BRANDMILLER J.C.- The G.I. factor : the glycaemic index solution. The scientific
answer to weight reduction and blood sugar control A Holder & Stroughton Book,
Australia, 1997

FONTVIEILLE A.M.- A moderate switch from high to low glycaemic-index foods for
3 weeks improves the metabolic control of type I diabetic subjects -
Diab.Nutr.Metab., 1988, 1, 139-143

JENKINS DJA Glycemic index of foods : a physiological basis for carbohydrate
exchange - Am.J.Clin.nutr., 1981, 34, 362-366

JENKINS DJA- Metabolic effects of low-glycemic index diet
Am.J.Clin.Nutr.1987, 46, 968-975

JENKINS DJA - Low glycemic index ; lente carbohydrates and physiological effects
of altered food frequency
Am.J.Clin.Nutr., 1994, 56 (suppl), 706 S-709 S

LORMEAU B., VALENSI P. - L'alimentation du diabétique Cah.Nutr.Diet., 1997, 32,
6, 394-400

MONNIER L., SLAMA G. -Recommandations ALFEDIAM
Diabetes Metabolism, 1995, 21, 201-217
Nutritional recommendations and principles for individuals with diabetes mellitus
Diabetes care, 1990, 13, suppl I, 18-25

O'DEA K. - Physical factors influency post-prandial glucose and insulin responses to
starch - Am.J.Clin.Nutr., 1980, 33, 760-765

SIMPSON HCR - A high carbohydrate leguminous fibre diet improves all aspects of
diabetic control- Lancet, 1981, 1, 1-5

SLAMA G. Diabete : conseils nutritionnels
Impact Médecin Hebdo, 13 Juin 1997, N°370, 51-53

PHYSICAL ACTIVITY & EXERCISE:

BLAIR D. Habitual daily energy expenditure and activity levels of lean and adult-onset and child-onset obese women
Am.J.Clin.Nutr., 1987, 45, 540-550

BLAIR S.N. Evidence for success of exercise in weight loss and control - Annals of Int.Med., 1993, 119, 7, 2 ; 702-706

DESPRES JP Obésité abdominale et lipoprotéines : effets de l'exercice - Science et Sports, 1991, 6, 265-273

DESPRES JP L'exercice physique dans le traitement de l'obésité Cah. Nutr. Diet., 1994, XXIX, 5, 299-304

GUEZENNEC CY - Place de l'entraînement dans le traitement des maladies métaboliques - Cah.Nutr.Diet., 1994, XXIX, 1, 28-37

KEMPEN KPG - Energy balance during an 8-weeks energy-restricted diet with and without exercice in obese women
Am.J.Clin.Nutr., 1995, 62, 722-729

LOUIS SYLVESTRE J. Insuline et exercice physique. Diabète et Métabolisme, 1987, 13, 152-156

MONDENARD de JP- Poids et sport. Précis de Nutrition et Diététique , Fasc. 17, Ardix Médical, 1989

MARCONNET P. Effort musculaire et substrats énergétiques Cah. Nutr. Diet., 1986, XXI, 2, 109-122

TREMBLAY A Exercice et obésité Science et Sports, 1991, 6, 257-264

WOLF LM Contribution de l'exercice physique au traitement de l'obésité - Cah.Nutr.Diet, 1986, XXI, 2, 137-141

WOOD PD The effects on plasqma lipoproteins of a prudent weight-reducing diet, with or without exercise, in overweight men and women - N.Engl.J.Med., 1991, 325, 461-466

HYPOGLYCEMIA:

CAHILL G.F. A non editorial on non hypoglycemia N. Engl. J. Med. 1974,291, 905-906

CATHELINEAU G. Effect of calcium infusion on post reactive hypoglycemia Horm. Meatb. Res. 1981,13, 646-647

CHILES R. Excessive serum insulin response to oral glucose in obesity and mild diabets Diabetes 1970,19.458

CRAPO P.A. The effects of oral fructose, sucrose and glucose in subjects with reactive hypoglycemia
Diabetes care 1982,5 ,512-517

DORNER M. Les hypoglycémies fonctionnelles Rev. Prat. 1972,22,25, 3427-3446

FAJANS S.S. Fasting hypoglycemia in adults New Engl. J. Med. 1976, 294, 766-772

FARRYKANT M. The problem of fonctionnal hyperinsulinism or fonctional hypoglycemia attributed to nervous causes
Metabolism 1971,20,6,428-434

FIELD J.B.Studies on the mechanisms of ethanol induced hypoglycemia J. Clin. Invest. 1963,42,497-506

FREINKEL N. Alcohol hypoglycemia J. Clin. Invest 1963,42,1112-1133

HARRIS S. Hyperinsulinism and dysinsulinism J.A.M.A. 1924, 83,729-733

HAUTECOUVERTURE M. Les hypoglycémies fonctionnelles Rev. Prat. 1985, 35, 31, 1901-1907

HOFELDT F.D. Reactive hypoglycemia Metab. 1975,24,1193-1208

HOFELDT F.D. Are abnormalities in insulin secretion responsable for reactive hypoglycemia ? Diabetes 1974,23,589-596

JENKINS D.J.A. Decrease in post-prandial insulin and glucose concentrations by guar and pectin
Ann. Intern. Med. 1977, 86, 20-23

JOHNSON D.D. Réactive hypoglycemia J.A.M.A. 1980, 243, 1151-1155

JUNG Y. Reactive hypoglycemia in women Diabetes 1971, 20,428-434

LEFEBVRE P. Statement on post-prandial hypoglycemia Diabetes care 1988, 11, 439-440

LEFEBVRE P. Le syndrome d'hypoglycémie réactionnelle, mythe ou réalité ?
Journées Annuelles de l'Hôtel-Dieu 1983, 111-118

LEICHTER S.B. Alimentary hypoglycemia: a new appraisal Amer. J. Nutr. 1979,32,2104-2114

LEV-RAN A. The diagnosis of post-prandial hypoglycemia Diabetes 1981, 30, 996-999

LUBETZKI J.Physiopathologie des hypoglycémies Rev. Prat. 1972, 22, 25, 3331-3347

LUYCKY A.S. Plasma insulin in reactive hypoglycemia Diabetes 1971, 20,435-442

MONNIER L.H. Restored synergistic entero-hormonal response after addition dietary fibre to patients with impaired glucose tolerance and reactive hypoglycemia Diab. Metab. 1982,8.217-222

O'KEEFE SJ.D. Lunch time gin and tonic: a cause of reactive hypoglycemia Lancet 1977, 1, June 18,1286-1288

PERRAULT M. Le régime de fond des hypoglycémies fonctionnelles de l'adulte Rev. Prat. 1963,13,4025-4030

SENG G. Mécanismes et conséquences des hypoglycémies Rev. Prat. 1985, 35, 31, 1859-1866

SERVICE J.F. Hypoglycemia and the post-prandial syndrom New Ene. J. Med. 1989,321,1472

SUSSMAN K.E. Plasma insulin levels during reactive hypoglycemia Diabetes 1966,15,1-14

TAMBURRANO G. Increased insulin sensitivity in patients with idiopathic reactive hypoglycemia
J. Clin. Endocr. Metab.,1989, 69, 885

TAYLOR S.I. Hypoglycemia associated with antibodies to the insulin receptor. New. Engl. J. Med. 1982,307. 1422-1426

YALOW R.S. Dynamics of insulin secretion in hypoglycemia Diabctes 1965, 14, 341-350

INDEX

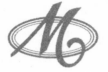